Pocket Guide to Physical Assessment

Pocket Guide to Physical Assessment

Edited by

Carol Lynn Cox

PhD, MSc, MA (Theology), MA (Education), PG Dip Education, BSc (Hons), RN, ENB 254, FHEA

Professor Emeritus, School of Health Sciences, City, University of London, London, UK and Clinical Manager and Director of Nursing, Health and Hope Clinics, Pensacola, FL, USA

Adapted from *Lecture Notes on Clinical Skills* (Third Edition) by:

The late Robert Turner MD, FRCP

Professor of Medicine and Honorary Consultant Physician Nuffield Department of Clinical Medicine Radcliffe Infirmary, Oxford, UK

Roger Blackwood MA, FRCP

Consultant Physician, Wexham Park Hospital, Slough, and Honorary Consultant Physician at Hammersmith Hospital, London, UK

WILEY Blackwell

Registered Office(s)
John Wiley & Sons, Inc., 111 River Street, Hoboken, NJ 07030, USA
John Wiley & Sons Ltd, The Atrium, Southern Gate, Chichester, West Sussex, PO19 8SQ, UK

Editorial Office
9600 Garsington Road, Oxford, OX4 2DQ, UK

For details of our global editorial offices, customer services, and more information about Wiley products visit us at www.wiley.com.

Wiley also publishes its books in a variety of electronic formats and by print-on-demand. Some content that appears in standard print versions of this book may not be available in other formats.

Library of Congress Cataloging-in-Publication Data
Names: Cox, Carol Lynn, editor. | Adaptation of (expression): Turner, Robert, 1938–1999. Lecture notes on clinical skills. 3rd edition.
Title: Pocket guide to physical assessment / edited by Carol Lynn Cox.
Description: Hoboken, NJ : Wiley-Blackwell, 2019. | Adapted from Lecture notes on clinical skills / Robert Turner, Roger Blackwood. 3rd ed. 1997. | Includes bibliographical references and index. |
Identifiers: LCCN 2019003275 (print) | LCCN 2019004179 (ebook) | ISBN 9781119108931 (Adobe PDF) | ISBN 9781119108948 (ePub) | ISBN 9781119108924 (pbk.)
Subjects: | MESH: Physical Examination–methods | Diagnostic Techniques and Procedures | Handbook
Classification: LCC RC78.7.D53 (ebook) | LCC RC78.7.D53 (print) | NLM WB 39 | DDC 616.07/54–dc23
LC record available at https://lccn.loc.gov/2019003275

Cover Design: Wiley
Cover Images: © George Doyle/Getty Images, © Seth Joel/Getty Images, © Jeffrey Coolidge/Getty Images, © kokouu/Getty Images

Set in 11.5/13.5pts STIX Two Text by SPi Global, Pondicherry, India
Printed and bound in Singapore by Markono Print Media Pte Ltd

10 9 8 7 6 5 4 3 2 1

Contents

List of Contributors

Graham M. Boswell, DEd, MA Ed, BA (Hons), BSc (Hons) RGN, FHEA
Senior Lecturer, Department of Adult Nursing and Paramedic Science, Faculty of Education and Health, University of Greenwich, London, UK

Carol Lynn Cox, PhD, MSc, MA (Theology), MA (Education), PG Dip Education, BSc (Hons), RN, ENB 254, FHEA
Professor Emeritus, School of Health Sciences, City, University of London, London, UK and Clinical Manager and Director of Nursing, Health and Hope Clinics, Pensacola, FL, USA

Helen Gibbons MSc, PG Cert (Medical Education), ENB (Ophthalmic Practice), BA (Hons), RN
Clinical Nursing Lead (Education and Research), Moorfields Eye Hospital NHS Foundation Trust and Course Director, University College London, London, UK

Victoria Lack, MSN, PG Dip (Academic Practice), BN (Hons), Family Nurse Practitioner, Non-Medical Prescriber, DN (Cert), RN
Lecturer in Primary Care, Department of Health Sciences, University of York, York, UK, and Advanced Nurse Practitioner, Beech House Surgery, Knaresborough, North Yorkshire, UK

Anthony McGrath, PhD, MSc, PGCE, BA (Hons) RMN, RGN, FHEA
Principal Lecturer, Head of Adult Nursing and Midwifery, London South Bank University, London, UK

Nicola L. Whiteing, PhD, MSc, PG Dip HE, BSc (Hons), RN, RNT, ANP
Lecturer in Nursing, Southern Cross University, New South Wales, Australia

Foreword

Underpinning the appropriate delivery of healthcare is the Physical Assessment. This structured physical examination allows the healthcare professional to obtain a comprehensive assessment of the patient and is critically important in that it leads to clinical decisions that are crucial for the patients' care.

This Pocket Book, *Pocket Guide to Physical Assessment*, provides a clear and easy-to-use reference guide for achieving the Physical Assessment. It is specifically intended for those embarking on a career in healthcare and contains the techniques used by specialist/advanced practitioners.

In this Pocket Guide, the need for a thorough approach to the Physical Assessment is excellently presented by Professor Cox. Professor Cox shows how important it is to develop a rapport with the patient in order to carefully assess their perceptions and how this relationship must be established from the very first meeting when information is exchanged between the healthcare professional and the patient. Fundamental to gaining this perspective is to listen. The importance of guiding the healthcare practitioner to engage in active listening cannot be underestimated and this is reflected in the fact that not being heard is an issue that is often raised as a point of criticism of healthcare professionals by patients and their families.

Careful observation and reports of subjective symptoms are the window through which healthcare professionals gain knowledge of their patients. Following the opening chapters, this Pocket Guide is structured to enable the healthcare professional to learn how to systematically gather information before moving on to an initial diagnosis and further investigations. The tools of inspection, palpation, percussion, and auscultation are key to this assessment and are excellently laid out in the chapters covering the examination of the different organs of the body.

It is key for healthcare professionals to be able to communicate the outcomes of their Physical Assessment to their professional colleagues. Professor Cox demonstrates her experience and understanding of the world of healthcare when she talks about the importance of this communication between professionals and how the Physical Assessment can bring together the disparate professional views that will underpin the diagnostic process.

In this *Pocket Guide to Physical Assessment*, Professor Cox has created an invaluable guide that will not only support practitioners as they begin a clinical career in healthcare but will also function as an ongoing reference book to support their careers.

Professor Stanton Newman, Pro Vice Chancellor Research,
City University London, England, UK

Preface

Over the past decade many changes have occurred in relation to medical practice. What has not changed, and should not change, is the view healthcare professionals have in relation to the patient. This view sees the patient as an individual with physical as well as emotional, psychological, intellectual, social, cultural, and spiritual needs. A comprehensive assessment of the patient is the foundation upon which healthcare decisions are made. The best way to develop assessment skills is to learn them systematically. The systematic approach involves taking a full health history, physical examination, and reviewing diagnostic texts/laboratory data. Use of a systematic approach is essential in clinical decision making, which leads to the formulation of a differential diagnosis and final diagnosis.

This Pocket Guide for healthcare professionals is based on Robert Turner's and Roger Blackwood's *Lecture Notes on Clincal Skills* that was written for medical students and Carol Cox's Physical Assessment for Nurses. It is intended to be used as a guide when examining patients in the clinical setting. The Guide includes simple instructions on examination approaches and details of diseases that are relevant to abnormal findings.

Turner and Blackwood's *Lecture Notes on Clinical Skills* has been used in the Oxford Clinical Medical School for over 35 years and is viewed as an essential guide in medicine. Although some doctors may use slightly different techniques in taking a history and physical examination, it is recommended that healthcare practitioners embarking on a career in healthcare use the techniques recommended in this Pocket Guide because they provide a sound approach for developing and employing clinical decision making.

Carol Lynn Cox

Acknowledgements

Special thanks are extended to Robert Turner and Roger Blackwood for granting permission for their text, *Lecture Notes on Clinical Skills*, to be used as a reference for this Pocket Guide. In addition, I am grateful to my students and healthcare practitioners that I have worked with over the years for encouraging me to create this Pocket Guide so that they could have an accessible tool for reference purposes in the clinical setting. This Guide has benefited from their suggestions as well as from medical colleagues with whom I currently practice. I am also grateful to Yogalakshmi Mohanakrishnan, Mitch Fitton, Copy Editor, Tom Marriott, Editorial Assistant, Vincent Rajan, Production Editor and the entire team at Wiley Publishers for their support in completing this Pocket Guide. Any faults or omissions in the text are entirely my own.

1

Interviewing and History Taking

Carol Lynn Cox[1,2]
[1] *School of Health Sciences, City, University of London, London, UK*
[2] *Health and Hope Clinics, Pensacola, FL, USA*

1.1 General Procedures

1.1.1 Introduction

The patient's history is the major subjective source of data about their health status. It will give you insight into actual and potential problems as well as providing a guide for the physical examination. History taking involves obtaining the patient's chief complaint (quoted in the patient's words), a full review of systems from the patient's perspective, exploration of patient problems associated with the chief complaint, and other (frequently associated) problems that require addressing from the patient's perspective (Ball et al. 2014a, b; Barkauskas et al. 2002; Bickley and Szilagyi 2007, 2013; Cox 2010; Dains et al. 2012, 2015; Epstein et al. 2008; Japp and Robertson 2013; Jarvis 2008, 2015; Seidel et al. 2006, 2010; Swartz 2006; Talley and O'Connor 2006, 2014).

Pocket Guide to Physical Assessment, First Edition. Edited by Carol Lynn Cox.

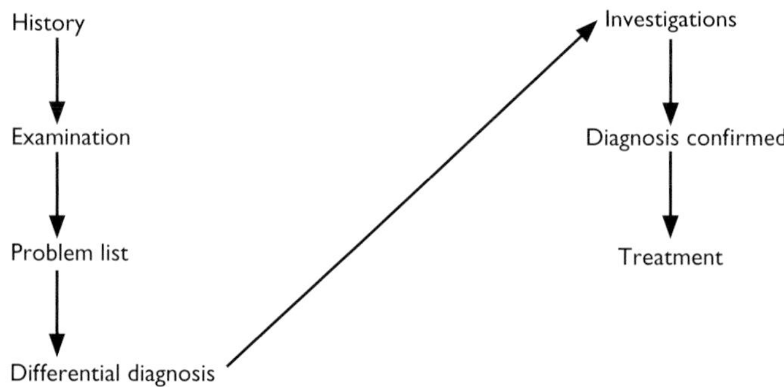

Figure 1.1 Usual sequence of events. Source: Cox 2010. Reproduced with permission from John Wiley and Sons.

1.1.2 Approaching the Patient

- Put the patient at ease by being confident and quietly friendly (Hatton and Blackwood 2003; Jackson and Vessey 2010; Rudolf and Levene 2011; Sawyer 2012).
- Greet the patient: 'Good morning, Mr/Mrs Smith'. (Address the patient formally and use the full name until the patient has given you permission for less formal address.)
- Shake the patient's hand or place your hand on theirs if the patient is ill. (This action begins your physical assessment. It will give you a baseline indication of the patient's physical condition. For example, cold, clammy, diaphoretic, or pyrexial.)
- State your name and title/role.
- Make sure the patient is comfortable.
- Explain that you wish to ask the patient questions to find out what the patient perceives is the problem or has happened.

  Start the history taking by stating something like 'I want to start by asking you some questions about your health'. (Always begin with general questions and then move to more specific questions (Cox 2010) Inform the patient how long you are likely to take and what to expect. For example, after discussing what has happened to the patient, explain that you would like to examine them.

1.1.3 Usual Sequence of Events (Figure 1.1)

1.1.3.1 Importance of the History

- It identifies:
    - what the problem is or has happened
    - the personality of the patient
    - how the illness has affected the patient and family
    - any specific anxieties
    - the physical and social environment.
- It establishes the practitioner–patient relationship.
- It provides the foundation for your differential diagnoses.
- It often gives the diagnosis.
- Find the principal symptoms or symptom. Ask one of the following questions:
    - 'How may I help you?'
    - 'What has the problem been?'
    - 'Tell me, why have you come to the surgery/clinic/hospital today?' or 'Tell me why you came to see me today?'

      Effective history taking involves allowing the patient to talk in an unstructured way whilst you maintain control of the interview. Use language that the patient can understand and avoid the use of medical jargon (Collins-Bride and Saxe 2013; Cox 2010; Sawyer 2012; Tally and O'Connor 2014). Avoid asking questions that can be answered by a simple 'yes' or 'no'. Ask questions that require a graded response. For example, 'Describe how your headache feels'. Avoid using multiple-choice questions that may confuse the patient (Cox 2010; Jackson and Vessey 2010). Ask one question at a time.

Avoid asking questions like: 'What's wrong?' or 'What brought you here?' Use clarification to confirm your understanding of the patient's problem. Avoid forming premature conclusions about the patient's problem and above all remain nonjudgemental in your demeanour. Avoid making judgemental statements.

- Let the patient tell their story in their own words as much as possible.

  At first listen and then take discreet notes as the patient talks.

  When learning to take a history there can be a tendency to ask too many questions in the first two minutes. After asking the first question you should normally allow the patient to talk uninterrupted for up to two minutes.

  Do not worry if the story is not entirely clear or if you do not think the information being given is of diagnostic significance. If you interrupt too early, you run the risk of overlooking an important symptom or anxiety.

  You will be learning about what the patient thinks is important. You have the opportunity to judge how you are going to proceed. Different patients give histories in very different ways. Some patients will need to be encouraged to enlarge on their answers to your questions; with other patients, you may need to ask specific questions and to interrupt in order to prevent too rambling a history. Think consciously about the approach you will adopt. If you need to interrupt the patient, do so clearly and decisively. Most important, do not give the impression you are in a hurry to conclude the discussion as this impression may cause the patient to withhold valuable information you need before commencing your physical examination.

- Try, if feasible, to conduct a conversation rather than an interrogation, following the patient's train of thought.
  You will usually need to ask follow-up questions on the main symptoms to obtain a full understanding of what they were and of the chain of events.
- Obtain a full description of the patient's principal complaints.
- Enquire about the sequence of symptoms and events. Beware pseudomedical terms, e.g. 'gastric flu' – enquire what happened. Clarify by asking what the patient means.
- Do not ask leading questions.
  A central aim in taking the history is to understand patients' symptoms from their own point of view. It is important not to tarnish the patient's history by your own expectations. For example, do not ask a patient whom you suspect might be thyrotoxic: 'Do you find hot weather uncomfortable?' This invites the answer 'yes' and then a positive answer becomes of little diagnostic value. Ask the open question: 'Do you particularly dislike either hot or cold weather?' (Ball et al. 2014a, b; Bickley and Szilagyi 2013; Coulehan 2006).
- Be sensitive to a patient's mood and nonverbal responses.
  For example, hesitancy in revealing emotional content. Use reflection so that the patient will expand on their discussion.
- Be understanding, receptive, and matter of fact without being sympathetic. Display and express empathy rather than sympathy.
- Avoid showing surprise or reproach.
- Clarify symptoms and obtain a problem list.
- When the patient has finished describing the symptom or symptoms:

- briefly summarise the symptoms
- ask whether there are any other main problems (Coulehan 2006).
  For example, say, 'You have mentioned two problems: pain on the left side of your tummy, and loose motions over the last six weeks. Before we talk about those in more detail, are there any other problems I should know about?'

1.1.4 Usual Sequence of History

- nature of principal complaints, e.g. chest pain, poor home circumstances
- history of present complaint
- details of current illness
- enquiry of other symptoms (see Functional Enquiry)
- past history
- family history
- personal and social history

- If one's initial enquiries make it apparent that one section is of more importance than usual (e.g. previous relevant illnesses or operation), then relevant enquiries can be brought forward to an earlier stage in the history (e.g. past history after finding principal complaints).

1.1.5 History of Present Illness

- Start your written history with a single sentence summing up what your patient's complaint is. It should be like the banner headline of a newspaper. For example: c/o chest pain for six months.
  (It is best to state in quotation marks the patient's chief complaint in the patient's own words when documenting.)

- Determine the chronology of the illness by asking:
    - 'How and when did your illness begin?' or
    - 'When did you first notice anything wrong?' or
    - 'When did you last feel completely well?'
- Begin by stating when the patient was last perfectly well. Describe symptoms in chronological order of onset.

  Both the date of onset and the length of time prior to being seen by you should be recorded. Symptoms should never be dated by the day of the week as this later becomes meaningless (Bickley and Szilagyi 2007, 2013; Cox 2010).
- Obtain a detailed description of each symptom by asking:
    - 'Tell me what the pain was like', for example. Make sure you ask about all symptoms, whether they seem relevant or not.
- With all symptoms obtain the following details:
    - duration
    - onset – sudden or gradual
    - what has happened since:
        - constant or periodic
        - frequency
        - getting worse or better
    - precipitating or relieving factors
    - associated symptoms.
- If pain is a symptom also determine the following:
    - site
    - radiation
    - character, e.g. ache, pressure, shooting, stabbing, dull
    - severity, e.g. 'Did it interfere with what you were doing?' 'Does it keep you awake?' 'Have you ever had this type of pain before?' 'Does the pain make you sweat or feel sick to your stomach?'

Avoid technical language when describing a patient's history. Do not say 'the patient complained of melaena', rather: 'the patient complained of passing loose, black, tarry motions'.

1.1.6 Supplementary History

When patients are unable to give an adequate or reliable history, the necessary information must be obtained from friends or relations. A history from a person who has witnessed a sudden event is often helpful.

When the patient does not speak English, arrange for an interpreter to translate for the patient. Bear in mind that numerous authors (Barkauskas et al. 2002; Ball et al. 2014a; Bickley and Szilagyi 2013; Cox 2010; Jarvis 2015; Rhoads and Paterson 2013) indicate that, if possible, family members and patients' young children should not be used as interpreters. Family members will frequently tell you what they think the patient's problem is rather than what the patient thinks the problem is. Because some questions that you may ask the patient are sensitive in nature, children should not be asked to interpret for their parents (Cox 2010; Lack 2012).

1.2 Functional Enquiry

This is a checklist of symptoms not already discovered.

Do not ask questions already covered in establishing the principal symptoms. This list may detect other symptoms.

- Modify your questioning according to the nature of the suspected disease, available time, and circumstances (Lack 2012).
  If during the functional enquiry a positive answer is obtained, full details must be elicited. **Asterisks (*) denote questions that must nearly always be asked.**

1.2.1 General Questions (These May Be Considered as Part of your Review of Systems)

- Ask about the following points:
    - *appetite: 'What is your appetite like? Do you feel like eating?'
    - *weight: 'Have you lost or gained weight recently?'
    - *general well-being: 'Do you feel well in yourself?'
    - *feelings of sadness or depression (to rule out feelings of suicide): 'Do you feel sad or depressed?'
    - fatigue: 'Are you more or less tired than you used to be?'
    - fever or chills: 'Have you felt hot or cold? Have you shivered?'
    - night sweats: 'Have you noticed any sweating at night or any other time?'
    - aches or pains
    - rash: 'Have you had any rash recently? Does it itch?'
    - lumps and bumps.

1.2.2 Cardiovascular and Respiratory System

- Ask about the following points:
    - *chest pain: 'Have you recently had any pain or discomfort in the chest?'

The most common causes of chest pain are:

- *ischaemic heart disease*: severe constricting, central chest pain radiating to the neck, jaw, and left arm; *angina*: pain frequently precipitated by exercise or emotion and relieved by rest; *myocardial infarction*; the pain may come on at rest, be more severe, and last hours

- *pleuritic pain*: sharp, localised pain, usually lateral; worse on inspiration or cough
- *anxiety or panic attacks*: a very common cause of chest pain. Enquire about circumstances that bring on an attack.
- *shortness of breath: 'Are you breathless at any time?'

Breathlessness (dyspnoea) and chest pain must be accurately described. The degree of exercise that brings on the symptoms must be noted (e.g. climbing one flight of stairs, after 0.5 km [1/4 mi] walk).

- shortness of breath on lying flat (*orthopnoea*): 'Do you get breathless in bed? What do you do then? Does it get worse or better on sitting up? How many pillows do you use? Can you sleep without them?'
- waking up breathless: 'Do you wake at night with any symptoms? Do you gasp for breath? What do you do then?'

Orthopnoea (breathless when lying flat) and *paroxysmal nocturnal dyspnoea* (waking up breathless, relieved on sitting up) are features of *left heart failure*.

- *ankle swelling

Common in *congestive cardiac failure* (*right heart failure*).

- palpitations: 'Are you aware of your heart beating?'

Palpitations may be:

- single thumps (*ectopics*)
- slow or fast
- regular or irregular

Ask the patient to tap them out.

Paroxysmal tachycardia (sudden attacks of palpitations) usually starts and finishes abruptly.

- *cough: ‘Do you have a cough? Is it a dry cough or do you cough up sputum? When do you cough?’
- sputum: ‘What colour is your sputum? How much do you cough up?’

Green sputum usually indicates an *acute chest infection.* Clear sputum daily during winter months suggests *chronic bronchitis.* Frothy sputum suggests *left heart failure.*

- *blood in sputum (*haemoptysis*): ‘Have you coughed up blood?’

Haemoptysis must be taken very seriously. Causes include:

- carcinoma of bronchus
- pulmonary embolism
- mitral stenosis
- tuberculosis
- bronchiectasis
- blackouts (*syncope*): ‘Have you had any blackouts or faints? Did you feel light-headed or did the room go round? Did you lose consciousness? Did you have any warning? Can you remember what happened?’
- *smoking: ‘Do you smoke? How many cigarettes do you smoke each day?’

1.2.3 Gastrointestinal System

- Ask about the following points:
  - nausea: ‘Are there times when you feel sick?’
  - vomiting: ‘Do you vomit? What is it like?’

'Coffee grounds' vomit suggests 'altered' blood such as with a bleeding ulcer.

Old food suggests *pyloric stenosis.*

If blood, what colour is it – dark or bright red?

- difficulty in swallowing (*dysphagia*): 'Do you have difficulty swallowing? Where does it stick?'

For solids: often organic obstruction.

For fluids: often neurological or psychological.

- indigestion: 'Do you have any discomfort in your stomach after eating?'
- abdominal pain: 'Where is the pain? How is it connected to meals or opening your bowels? What relieves the pain?'
- *bowel habit: 'How often do you open your bowels?' or 'How many times do you open your bowels per day?' 'Do you have to open your bowels at night?' (often a sign of true pathology)

If *diarrhoea* is suggested, the number of motions per day and their nature (blood? pus? mucus?) must be established. Frothy, frequent diarrhoea may be suggestive of coeliac disease.

'What are your motions like?' The stools may be pale, bulky, and float (fat in stool – *steatorrhoea*) or tarry from digested blood (*melaena* – usually from upper gastrointestinal tract).

Bright blood on the surface of a motion may be from *haemorrhoids*, whereas blood in a stool may signify *cancer* or *inflammatory bowel disease.*

Question what the patient has eaten. Red stool may indicate the patient has been eating beets, for example.

- jaundice: 'Is your urine dark? Are your stools pale? What tablets have you been taking recently? Have you had any recent injections or transfusions? Have you been abroad recently? How much alcohol do you drink?'

Jaundice may be:

- obstructive (dark urine, pale stools) from:
  - carcinoma of the head of the pancreas
  - gallstones
- hepatocellular (dark urine, pale stools may develop) from:
  - *ethanol* (cirrhosis)
  - drugs or transfusions (viral hepatitis)
  - drug reactions or infections (travel abroad, viral hepatitis, or amoebae)
- haemolytic (unconjugated bilirubin is bound to albumin and is not secreted in the urine).

1.2.4 Genitourinary System

- Ask about the following points:
  - dysuria: pain on urination – usually burning (often a sign of infection/cystitis)
  - loin pain: 'Any pain in your back?'

Pain in the loins suggests pyelonephritis.

- *urine: 'Are your waterworks all right? Do you pass a lot of water at night? Do you have any difficulty passing water? Is there blood in your water?' (suggests haematuria)

Polyuria and *nocturia* occur in *diabetes*.

Prostatism results in slow onset of urination, a poor stream, and terminal dribbling.

- sex: 'Any problems with intercourse or making love?'
- *menstruation: 'Any problems with your periods? Do you bleed heavily? Do you bleed between periods?'

Vaginal bleeding between periods or after the menopause raises the possibility of *cervical* or *uterine cancer*.

Menstrual cycle: Last menstrual period (**LMP**) and length of bleeding. (Normal cycle is 21–35 days. Normal period is between 5 and 8 days with between 70 and 200 ml of blood loss.) If indicated, ask about intermenstrual bleeding, postmenopausal bleeding or postcoital bleeding.

- vaginal discharge (if present, ask about colour, consistency, and odour; does it cause itching?)
- pain on intercourse (*dyspareunia*).

1.2.5 Nervous System

- Ask about the following points:
  - *headache: 'Do you ever have any headaches? Where are they?' (location) 'When do you get headaches?' 'What are they like?' (quality/intensity)

Headaches often originate from tension and can be either frontal or occipital. Occipital headache on waking in the early morning may be due to *raised intracranial pressure* (e.g. from a *tumour* or *malignant hypertension*). Ask if the headache is associated with flashing lights (*amaurosis fugax*) (Bickley and Szilagyi 2013; Cox 2010).

- vision: 'Do you have any blurred or double vision?'
- hearing: ask about tinnitus, deafness, and exposure to noise
- dizziness: 'Do you have any dizziness or episodes when the world goes round (*vertigo*)?'

Dizziness with light-headed symptoms, when sudden in onset, may be *cardiac* (enquire about palpitations). When slow, onset may be *vasovagal 'fainting'* or an *internal haemorrhage.*

Vertigo may be from ear disease *(labyrinthitis/infection, Ménière's disease, Benign Paroxysmal Positional Vertigo [BPPV] 'Ear Crystals' and/or age related)*

Enquire about deafness, earache, or discharge or *brainstem dysfunction.*

- unsteady gait: 'Any difficulty walking or running?'
- weakness (consider myelinating encephalophy [**ME**] or *myasthenia gravis*)
- numbness or increased sensation: 'Any patches of numbness?'
- pins and needles
- sphincter disturbance: 'Any difficulties holding your water/bowels?' (sign of spinal cord compression; ask about back injury)
- Fits or faints: 'Have you had any funny episodes?' (*Syncope – consider cardiac related*, e.g. *postural orthostatic tachycardia syndrome [POTS] – disautonomia*)

The following details should be sought from the patient:

- duration
- frequency and length of attacks
- time of attacks, e.g. if standing, at night
- mode of onset and termination
- premonition or aura, light-headedness, or vertigo
- biting of tongue, loss of sphincter control, injury, etc.

Grand mal epilepsy classically produces sudden unconsciousness without any warning and on waking the patient feels drowsy with a headache, has a sore tongue, and has been incontinent.

1.2.6 Mental Health

- Ask about the following points:
  - depression: 'How is your mood? Happy or sad? If depressed, how bad? Have you lost interest in things? Can you still enjoy things? How do you feel about the future?' 'Has anything happened in your life to make you sad or depressed? Do you feel guilty about anything?' If the patient seems depressed: 'Have you ever thought of suicide? How long have you felt like this? Is there a specific problem? Have you felt like this before?'
  - active periods: 'Do you have periods in which you are particularly active?'

Susceptibility to depression may be a personality trait. In *bipolar affective disorder*, swings to *mania* (excess activity, rapid speech, and excitable mood) can recur. Enquire about interest, concentration, irritability, sleep difficulties.

In schizophrenia active periods are associated with paranoia (*in conjunction with bipolar affective disorder the term is schizoaffective disorder*)

- anxiety: 'Have you worried a lot recently? Do you get anxious? In what situations? Are there any situations you avoid because you feel anxious?' 'Do you worry about your health? Any worries in your job or with your family? Any financial worries?' 'Do you have panic attacks? What happens?'
- sleep: 'Any difficulties sleeping? Do you have difficulty getting to sleep? Do you wake early?'

Difficulties of sleep are commonly associated with depression or anxiety.

In schizoaffective disorder both bipolar and schizophrenic behaviours are exhibited.

1.2.7 The Eye

- Ask about the following points:
    - eye pain, photophobia, or redness: 'Have the eyes been red, uncomfortable, or painful?'
    - painful red eye, particularly with photophobia, may be serious and due to:
      iritis (uveitis) – anterior/posterior uveitis must be treated as a medical emergency (it may be related to *ankylosing spondylitis, Reiter's disease, sarcoid, Behçet's disease. Uveitis is also seen in conjunction with ulcerative colitis and Crohn's disease.*)
        - *scleritis (systemic vasculitis)*
        - *corneal ulcer*
        - *acute glaucoma*
    - painless red eye may be:
      episcleritis
        - temporary and of no consequence
        - *systemic vasculitis*
    - sticky red eye may be *conjunctivitis* (usually infective)
    - itchy watery eye may be *allergic*, e.g. *hay fever*
    - gritty eye may be dry (sicca or *Sjögren's syndrome*)
    - clarity of vision: 'Has your vision been blurred?'
    - blurring of vision for either near or distance alone may be an error of focus, helped by spectacles
    - blurred vision in general (*serous retinopathy*)
    - loss of central vision (or of top or bottom half) in one eye may be due to a *retinal or optic nerve disorder*

- transient complete blindness in one eye lasting for minutes – *amaurosis fugax* (fleeting blindness) suggests retinal arterial blockage from embolus
    - may be from *carotid atheroma* (listen for bruit)
    - may have a cardiac source
- subtle difficulties with vision, difficulty reading – problems at the chiasm, or visual path behind it:
  complete *bitemporal hemianopia – tumour* pressure on chiasm
    - *homonymous*
    - *hemianopia*: *posterior cerebral* or *optic radiation lesion*
- usually *infarct* or *tumour*; rarely complains of 'half vision', but may have difficulty reading
- Diplopia: 'Have you ever seen double?'
- Diplopia may be due to:
    - *lesion* of the motor cranial nerves III, IV, or VI
    - *3rd-nerve palsy*

  causes double vision in all directions often with dilatation of the pupil and ptosis
    - *4th-nerve palsy*

  causes doubling looking down and in (as when reading) with images separated horizontally and vertically and tilted (not parallel)
    - *6th-nerve palsy*

  causes horizontal, level, and parallel doubling worse on looking to the affected side
    - *muscular disorder*

  e.g. thyroid related (see below)
  ME (weakness after muscle use, antibodies to nerve end plates)

Refer to Chapter 10 for more comprehensive information on examination of the eye.

1.2.8 Musculoskeletal System

- Ask about the following points:
  - pain, stiffness, or swelling of joints: 'When and how did it start? Have you injured the joint?' There are innumerable causes of *arthritis* (painful, swollen, tender joints) and *arthralgia* (painful joints). Patients may incorrectly attribute a problem to some injury.

    Osteoarthritis is a joint 'wearing out' and is often asymmetric, involving weight-bearing joints such as the hip or knee. Exercise makes the joint pain worse.

    Rheumatoid arthritis is a generalised autoimmune disease with symmetrical involvement. In the hands, fusiform swelling of the interphalangeal joints is accompanied by swollen metacarpophalangeal joints. Large joints are often affected. Stiffness is worse after rest, e.g. on waking, and improves with use.

    Gout usually involves a single joint, such as the first metatarsophalangeal joint, but can lead to gross hand involvement (also seen in the elbows and ankles) with asymmetric uric acid lumps (*tophi*) by some joints and in the tips of the ears.

    Septic arthritis is a single, hot, painful joint.
  - functional disability: 'How far can you walk? Can you walk up stairs? Is any particular movement difficult? Can you dress yourself? (Observe how the patient is dressed.) How long does it take?' 'Are you able to work?' 'Can you write?' (In the physical examination observe how the patient walks and their manual dexterity.)

Refer to Chapter 11 for more comprehensive information on examination of the musculoskeletal system.

1.2.9 Thyroid Disease

- Ask about the following points:
  - weight change
  - reaction to the weather: 'Do you dislike the hot or cold weather?'
  - irritability: 'Are you more or less irritable compared with a few years ago?'
  - diarrhoea/constipation
  - palpitations
  - dry skin or greasy hair: 'Is your skin dry or greasy? Is your hair dry or greasy?'
  - depression: 'How has your mood been?'
  - croaky voice

  Hypothyroid patients put on weight without increase in appetite; dislike cold weather; have dry skin and thin, dry hair, a puffy face, a croaky voice; are usually calm; and may be depressed.

  Hyperthyroid patients may lose weight despite eating more, dislike hot weather, perspire excessively, have palpitations and a tremor, and may be agitated and tearful. Young people have predominantly nervous and heat intolerance symptoms, whereas old people tend to present with cardiac symptoms. (Exophthalmos may be present.)

1.3 Past History

- All previous illnesses or operations, whether apparently important or not, must be included.
  For instance, a casually mentioned attack of influenza or chill may have been a manifestation of an occult infection.
- The importance of a past illness may be gained by finding out how long the patient was in bed or off work (Lack 2012).

- Complications of any previous illnesses should be carefully enquired into and, here, leading questions are sometimes necessary.

1.3.1 General Questions

- Ask about the following:
  - 'Have you had any serious illnesses?'
  - 'Have you had any emotional or nervous problems?'
  - 'Have you had any operations or admissions to hospital?'
  - 'Have you ever:
    - had yellow skin (jaundice), fits (epilepsy), tuberculosis, high blood pressure (hypertension), low blood pressure (hypotension), rheumatic fever, kidney problems, or diabetes?
    - travelled abroad?
    - had allergies?'
  - 'Have any medicines ever upset you?' Allergic responses to drugs may include an itchy rash, vomiting, diarrhoea, or severe illness, including jaundice. Many patients claim to be allergic but are not. An accurate description of the supposed allergic episodes is important.
  - Other questions can be included when relevant such as:
    - 'Have you ever had a heart attack?'
  - Additional questions can be asked depending on the patient's previous responses such as:
    - if the patient has high blood pressure, ask about kidney problems, if relatives have hypertension, or whether the patient eats liquorice

        - if a possible heart attack, ask about hypertension, diabetes, diet, smoking, family history of heart disease
        - if the history suggests cardiac failure, you must ask if the patient has had *rheumatic fever*

        Patients have often had examinations for life insurance, disability insurance, or the armed forces.

1.4 Family History

The family history gives clues to possible predisposition to illness (e.g. heart attacks) and whether a patient may have reason to be particularly anxious about a certain disease (e.g. mother died of cancer).

Death certificates and patient knowledge are often inaccurate. Patients may be reluctant to talk about relatives' illnesses if they were mental disorders, epilepsy, or cancer (Cox 2010).

It will be useful to construct a genogram of the patient's family history for quick referral.

1.4.1 General Questions

- Ask about the following:
    - 'Are your parents alive? Are they fit and well? What did your parents die from?'
    - 'Have you any brothers or sisters? Are they fit and well?'
    - 'Do you have any children? Are they fit and well?'
    - 'Is there any family history of:
        - heart trouble?
        - diabetes?
        - high blood pressure?'

These questions can be varied to take account of the patient's chief complaint.

1.5 Personal and Social History

You need to find out what kind of person the patient is, what their home circumstances are, and how the illness has affected the patient and family. Your aim is to understand the patient's illness in the context of their personality and home environment.

If in hospital or following day surgery, can the patient convalesce satisfactorily at home and at what stage? What are the consequences of the illness? Will advice, information, and help be needed? An interview with a relative or friend may be very helpful.

1.5.1 General Questions

- Ask about the following:
  - family: 'Is everything all right at home? Do you have any family problems?'
    It may be appropriate to ask: 'Is your relationship with your partner/husband/wife all right? Is sex all right?' Problems may arise from physical or emotional reasons, and the patient may appreciate an opportunity to discuss worries. Note that a patient's sexual preference and sexual orientation may be different.
  - accommodation: 'Where do you live? Is it all right?'
  - job: 'What is your job? Could you tell me exactly what you do? Is it satisfactory? Will your illness affect your work?'
  - hobbies: 'What do you do in your spare time? Do you have any social life?' 'What is your social life like?'
  - alcohol: 'How much alcohol do you drink?'

Alcoholics usually underestimate their daily consumption. (Normally intake should not exceed 21 units per week for a male and 14 units per week for a female.) It may be helpful to go through a 'drinking day'. If there is a suspicion of a drinking problem, you can ask: 'Do you ever drink in the morning? Do you worry about controlling your drinking? Does it affect your job, home, or social life?'

- smoking: 'Do you smoke?' Have you ever smoked? Why did you give up? How many cigarettes, e-ciagrettes (vapes, juuls, hookah pens) cigars, or pipefuls of tobacco do you smoke a day?'
  This is particularly relevant for heart or chest disease but must always be asked.
  (You may also consider asking about chewing tobacco in relation to mouth cancer.)
- drugs: 'Do you take any recreational drugs?' If so, 'What do you take?'
- prescribed medications: 'What pills (tablets) are you taking at the moment? Have you taken any other pills in the last few months?'

This is an extremely important question. A complete list of all drugs and doses must be obtained including complementary/integrative medicines and vitamins.

- If relevant, ask about any pets, visits abroad, previous or present exposure during working to coal dust, asbestos, etc.

1.5.2 The Patient's Ideas, Concerns, and Expectations

Make sure that you understand the patient's main ideas, concerns, and expectations. Ask for example:

- What do you think is wrong with you?
- What are you expecting to happen to you whilst you are in the surgery, clinic, or hospital?
- Is there something in particular you would like us to do?
- Have you any questions?

  The patient's main concerns may not be your main concerns. The patient may have quite different expectations of the visit to the surgery, the hospital admission, or outpatient appointment from what you assume. If you fail to address the patient's concerns they are likely to be dissatisfied, leading to a difficult practitioner–patient relationship and possible noncompliance (Coulehan 2006; Cox 2010).

1.5.3 Strategy

Having taken the history, you should:

- have some idea of possible diagnoses (in 90–95% of cases the patient will tell you what the problem is whilst you are taking the history)
- have made an assessment of the patient as a person
- know which systems you wish to concentrate on when examining the patient (Swartz 2014).

Further relevant questions may arise from abnormalities found on examination or investigation.

References

Ball, J., Dains, J., Flynn, J. et al. (2014a). *Seidel's Guide to Physical Examination*, 8e. St. Louis: Mosby.

Ball, J., Dains, J., Flynn, J. et al. (2014b). *Student Laboratory Manual to Accompany Seidel's Guide to Physical Examination*, 8e. St. Louis: Mosby.

Barkauskas, V., Baumann, L., and Darling-Fisher, C. (2002). *Health and Physical Assessment*, 3e. London: Mosby.

Bickley, L. and Szilagyi, P. (2007). *Bates' Guide to Physical Examination and History Taking*, 9e. Philadelphia: Lippincott.

Bickley, L. and Szilagyi, P. (2013). *Bates' Guide to Physical Examination and History Taking*, 11e. New York: Wolters Kluwer/Lippincott Williams & Wilkins.

Collins-Bride, G. and Saxe, J. (2013). *Clinical Guidelines for Advanced Practice Nursing – An Interdisciplinary Approach*, 2e. Burlington, MA: Jones and Bartlett Learning.

Coulehan, J. (2006). *The Medical Interview: Mastering Kills for Clinical Practice*, 5e. Philadelphia: F. A. David Company.

Cox, C. (2010). *Physical Assessment for Nurses*, 2e. Oxford: Wiley Blackwell.

Dains, J., Baumann, L., and Scheibel, P. (2012). *Advanced Health Assessment and Clinical Diagnosis in Primary Care*, 4e. St. Louis: Elsevier.

Dains, J., Baumann, L., and Scheibel, P. (2015). *Advanced Health Assessment and Clinical Diagnosis in Primary Care*, 5e. St. Louis: Mosby.

Epstein, O., Perkin, G., de Bono, D., and Cookson, J. (2008). *Clinical Examination*, 4e. London: Mosby.

Hatton, C. and Blackwood, R. (2003). *Lecture Notes on Clinical Skills*, 4e. Oxford: Blackwell Science.

Jackson, P. and Vessey, J. (2010). *Primary Care of the Child with a Chronic Condition*, 5e. London: Mosby.

Japp, A. and Robertson, C. (2013). *Macleod's Clinical Diagnosis.* Edinburgh: Churchill Livingstone, Elsevier.

Jarvis, C. (2008). *Physical Examination and Health Assessment*, 5e. St. Louis: Saunders.

Jarvis, C. (2015). *Physical Examination and Health Assessment*, 7e. Edinburgh: Elsevier.

Lack, V. (2012). Consultation skills. In: *Advanced Practice in Healthcare* (ed. C. Cox, M. Hill and V. Lack), 39–55. London: Routledge.

Rhoads, J. and Paterson, S. (2013). *Advanced Health Assessment and Diagnostic Reasoning*, 2e. Burlington: Jones and Bartlett.

Rudolf, M. and Levene, M. (2011). *Paediatrics and Child Health*, 3e. Oxford: Blackwell.

Sawyer, S.S. (2012). *Pediatric Physical Examination and Health Assessment*. London: Jones and Bartlett Learning International.

Seidel, H., Ball, J., Dains, J., and Benedict, G. (2006). *Mosby's Physical Examination Handbook*. St. Louis: Mosby.

Seidel, H., Ball, J., Dains, J., and Benedict, G. (2010). *Mosby's Physical Examination Handbook*, 7e. St. Louis: Mosby-Year Book.

Swartz, M. (2006). *Physical Diagnosis, History and Examination*, 5e. London: W. B. Saunders.

Swartz, M. (2014). *Physical Diagnosis: History and Examination*, With Student Consult Online Access, 7e. London: Elsevier.

Talley, N. and O'Connor, S. (2006). *Clinical Examination: A Systematic Guide to Physical Diagnosis*, 5e. London: Churchill Livingstone.

Talley, N. and O'Connor, S. (2014). *Clinical Examination: A Systematic Guide to Physical Diagnosis*, 7e. London: Churchill Livingstone, Elsevier.

2 General Health Assessment

Carol Lynn Cox[1,2]
[1] *School of Health Sciences, City, University University of London, London, UK*
[2] *Health and Hope Clinics, Pensacola, FL, USA*

2.1 Introduction

An initial assessment of the patient will have been made whilst taking the history. As a reminder, the history begins with the subjective component (patient's perspective) of your assessment, which includes a review of systems. The general appearance of the patient will be your first observation (Collins-Bride and Saxe 2013; Coulehan 2006; Hatton and Blackwood 2003; Lack 2012). Subsequently, the order of your physical examination will vary based on the subjective information provided in the patient's history. In an ideal world you would undertake your assessment following the Subjective, Objective, Assessment, and Plan (SOAP) format (Cox 2010). The SOAP format incorporates the subjective (chief complaint or presenting problem) from the patient's perspective, the objective examination you undertake, the assessment from the subjective and objective which is your impression of findings, your differential diagnosis, and finally your plan for the patient such as blood tests, X-rays, or other tests you want to order for the patient as

Pocket Guide to Physical Assessment, First Edition. Edited by Carol Lynn Cox.

well as instructions for the patient to follow including administration of medications and other treatments.

The system to which the presenting symptoms refer is generally examined first. Otherwise devise your own routine, examining each part of the body in turn, covering all systems as required. An example is:

- general appearance
- alertness, mood, general behaviour
- hands and nails
- skin
- radial pulse
- axillary nodes
- cervical lymph nodes
- facies, eyes, tongue
- jugular venous pulse/distension
- heart
- breasts
- respiratory
- abdomen, including femoral pulses
- rectal or pelvic examination
- musculoskeletal
- nervous system including fundi (if not examined with the eyes as noted above).

Whichever part of the body you are examining, always use the same routine*:

1. inspection
2. palpation
3. percussion
4. auscultation.

(*The routine will vary in examination of the abdomen with auscultation following inspection.) (Ball et al. 2014a, b; Barkauskas et al. 2002; Bickley and Szilagyi 2007, 2013; Cox 2010; Dains et al. 2015; Rundio and Lorman 2017)

2.2 General Inspection

The beginning of the examination is a careful observation of the patient as a whole. Note the following:

- Does the patient look ill?
    - what age does the patient look?
    - febrile, dehydrated?
    - alert, confused, drowsy?
    - cooperative, happy, sad, resentful?
    - obese, muscular, wasted?
    - in pain or distressed?

2.3 Hands

Note the following:

- Temperature:
    - unduly cold hands –? *low cardiac output*
    - unduly warm hands –? *high-output state*, e.g. *thyrotoxicosis*
    - cold and sweaty –? anxiety or other causes of *sympathetic overreactivity*, e.g. *hypoglycaemia*
- Peripheral cyanosis
- Raynaud's
- Nicotine stains
- Nails:
    - bitten
    - leukonychia – white nails
      Can occur in *cirrhosis*.
    - koilonychia – misshapen, concave nails
      Can occur in *iron-deficiency anaemia*.
    - clubbing – loss of angle at base of nail
      Nail clubbing occurs in specific diseases:
        - heart: infectious *endocarditis, cyanotic congenital heart disease*

        - lungs: *carcinoma of the bronchus* (*chronic infection*: *abscess*; *bronchiectasis*, e.g. *cystic fibrosis*; *empyema*); *fibrosing alveolitis* (not chronic bronchitis)
        - liver: *cirrhosis*
        - *Crohn's disease*
        - *congenital.*
    - splinter haemorrhages
      Occur in *infectious endocarditis* but are more common in people doing manual work.
    - pitting – *psoriasis*
    - onycholysis – separation of nail from nail bed; *psoriasis, thyrotoxicosis*
    - paronychia – pustule in lateral nail fold (Bickley and Szilagyi 2013; Collins-Bride and Saxe 2013; Dains et al. 2012, 2015; Epstein et al. 2008; Japp and Robertson 2013; Jarvis 2008).
- Palms:
    - erythema – can be normal, also occurs with *chronic liver disease, pregnancy*
    - Dupuytren's contracture – tethering of skin in palm to flexor tendon of fourth finger; can occur in *cirrhosis* (Barkauskas et al. 2002; Bickley and Szilagyi 2013; Collins-Bride and Saxe 2013; Dains et al. 2012, 2015; Jarvis 2008; Rundio and Lorman 2017; Seidel et al. 2006, 2010; Swartz 2006, 2014; Tally and O'Connor 2006, 2014).
- Joints:
    - symmetrical swellings occur in *rheumatoid arthritis*
    - asymmetrical swellings occur in *gout* and *osteoarthritis* (Bickley and Szilagyi 2013; Collins-Bride and Saxe 2013; Dains et al. 2012, 2015; Jarvis 2008; Rundio and Lorman 2017).

2.4 Skin

2.4.1 Inspection

- distribution of any lesions
- examine close up with palpation of skin
- remember mucous membranes, hair, and nails
- Colour:
    - pigmented apart from racial pigmentation or suntan – examine buccal mucosa
    - if appears jaundiced examine sclera
    - if pale examine conjunctivae for anaemia (if haemoglobin is less than 9 the conjunctivae will be pale to white)
- Skin texture:
    - ? normal for age (becomes thinner from age 50)
    - thin, e.g. *Cushing's syndrome, hypothyroid, hypopituitary, malnutrition, liver or renal failure*
    - thick, e.g. *acromegaly, androgen excess*
    - dry, e.g. *hypothyroid*
    - tethered or puckered, e.g. *scleroderma* of fingers, attached to underlying breast tumour
- Rash:
    - what is it like? (describe precisely)

2.4.2 Inspection of Lesions

- distribution of lesions:
  symmetrical or asymmetrical
  peripheral or mainly on trunk
  maximal on light-exposed sites
  pattern of contact with known agents, e.g. shoes, gloves, cosmetics
- number and size of lesions
- look at an early lesion
- discrete or confluent

- pattern of lesions, e.g. linear, annular, serpiginous (like a snake), reticular (like a net), star shaped (melanoma)
- is edge well demarcated? (Edges are well demarcated in syphilis for example.)
- colour (melanomas have atypical pigmentation in the epidermis such as shades of grey, white, red, blue, brown, and black)
- surface, e.g. scaly as in psoriasis; shiny as in thyrotoxicosis or peripheral vascular disease (Bickley and Szilagyi 2013; Collins-Bride and Saxe 2013; Dains et al. 2012, 2015; Jarvis 2008; Rundio and Lorman 2017; Tally and O'Connor 2014).

2.4.3 Palpation of Lesions

- flat, impalpable – *macular*
- raised
  papular: in skin, localised
  plaque: larger, e.g. > 0.5 cm
  nodules: deeper in dermis, persisting more than three days
  wheal: oedema fluid, transient, less than three days
  vesicles: contain fluid
  bullae: large vesicles, e.g. > 0.5 cm
  pustular
- deep in dermis – *nodules*
- temperature
- tender?
- blanches on pressure – most erythematous lesions, e.g. *drug rash, telangiectasia*, dilated capillaries
- does not blanch on pressure
  Purpura or *petechiae* are small discrete microhaemorrhages approximately 1 mm across, red, non-tender macules.
  If palpable, suggests *vasculitis.*

Senile purpura local haemorrhages are from minor traumas in thin skin of hands or forearms. Flat purple/brown lesions.

- hard
    - sclerosis, e.g. *scleroderma* of fingers
    - infiltration, e.g. *lymphoma* or *cancer*
    - scars (Japp and Robertson 2013; Jarvis 2015; Swartz 2014).

2.4.4 Enquire About the Time Course of any Lesion

- 'How long has it been there?'
- 'Is it fixed in size and position? Does it come and go?'
- 'Is it itchy, sore, tender or has no feeling (anaesthetic)?'

  Knowledge of the differential diagnosis will indicate other questions:

  dermatitis of hand – contact with chemicals or plants, wear and tear;

  ulcer of toe – arterial disease, diabetes mellitus, neuropathy;

  pigmentation and ulcer of lower medial leg – varicose veins.

2.4.5 Common Diseases

Acne	Pilar-sebaceous follicular inflammation – papules and pustules on face and upper trunk, blackheads (*comedones*), cysts.
Basal cell carcinoma (rodent ulcer)	Shiny papule with rolled border and capillaries on surface. Can have a depressed centre or ulcerate.
Bullae	Blisters due to burns, infection of the skin, allergy, or, rarely, autoimmune diseases affecting adhesion within epidermis (*pemphigus*) or at the epidermal–dermal junction (*pemphigoid*).

Café-au-lait patches

Permanent discrete brown macules of varying size and shape. If large and numerous (6 or>6 café-au-lait spots) requires evaluation – suggests neurofibromatosis.

Drug eruptions

Usually macular, symmetrical distribution. Can be urticaria, eczematous, and various forms, including erythema multiforme or erythema nodosum (see below).

Eczema

Atopic dermatitis: dry skin, red, plaques, commonly on the face, antecubital and popliteal fossae, with fine scales, vesicles, and scratch marks secondary to *pruritus* (itching).

Often associated with *asthma* and *hay fever.*

Family history of atopy.

Contact dermatitis: may be irritant or allergic.

Red, scaly plaques with vesicles in acute stages.

Erythema multiforme

Symmetrical, widespread inflammatory 0.5–1 cm macules/papules, often with central blister. Can be confluent. Usually on hands and feet:

drug reactions

viral infections

no apparent cause

Stevens–Johnson syndrome – with mucosal desquamation involving genitalia, mouth, and conjunctivae, with fever.

Erythema nodosum

Tender, localised, red, diffusely raised, 2–4 cm nodules in anterior shins. Due to:

streptococcal infection, e.g. with *rheumatic*

fever

primary tuberculosis and other infections

	sarcoid
	inflammatory bowel disease
	drug reactions
	no apparent cause
Fungus	Red, annular, scaly area of skin. When involving the nails, they become thickened with loss of compact structure.
Herpes infection	Clusters of vesicopustules which crust, recurs at the same site, e.g. lips, buttocks.
Impetigo	Spreading pustules and yellow crusts from staphylococcal infection.
Malignant melanoma	Usually irregular pigmented (grey, white, red, blue, brown, and black), papule or plaque, superficial or thick with irregular edge, enlarging with tendency to bleed.
Psoriasis	Symmetrical eruption: chronic, discrete, red plaques with silvery scales. Gentle scraping easily induces bleeding. Often affects scalp, elbows, and knees (may in severe cases cover the majority of the body). Nails may be pitted.
	Familial and precipitated by streptococcal sore throats or skin trauma.
Scabies	Mite infection: itching with 2–4 mm tunnels in epidermis, e.g. in webs of fingers, wrists, genitalia.
Squamous cell carcinoma	Warty localised thickening, may ulcerate.
Urticaria	Transient wheal with surrounding erythema. Lasts around 24 hours. Usually due to allergy to food or drugs, e.g. aspirin, or physical, e.g. dermographism, cold.
Vitiligo	Permanent demarcated, depigmented white patches due to autoimmune disease (Rundio and Lorman 2017).

2.5 Mouth

- Look at the tongue:
  - cyanosed, moist or dry

    Cyanosis is a reduction in the oxygenation of the blood, with more than 5 g dl^{-1} deoxygenated haemoglobin.

    Central cyanosis (blue tongue) denotes a right-to-left shunt (unsaturated blood appearing in systemic circulation):
    - congenital heart disease, e.g. *Fallot's tetralogy*
    - lung disease, e.g. *obstructive airways disease.*

    Peripheral cyanosis (blue fingers, pink tongue) denotes inadequate peripheral circulation.

    A dry tongue can mean salt and water deficiency (often called 'dehydration') but also occurs with mouth-breathing.
- Look at the teeth:
  - caries (exposed dentine), poor dental hygiene, false
- Look at the gums:
  - bleeding, swollen
- Look at the throat:
  - tonsils
  - pharynx: swelling, redness, ulceration
- Smell patient's breath:
  - ketosis (as in diabetes)
  - alcohol
  - foetor

    constipation, appendicitis

    musty in liver failure

  Ketosis is a sweet-smelling breath occurring with *starvation* or *severe diabetes.*

  Hepatic foetor is a musty smell in *liver failure* (Bickley and Szilagyi 2013; Collins-Bride and Saxe

2013; Dains et al. 2012, 2015; Jarvis 2008; Rundio and Lorman 2017; Tally and O'Connor 2014).

2.6 Eyes

Look at the eyes:

- *sclera*, icterus
  The most obvious demonstration of *jaundice* is the yellow sclera.
- lower lid conjunctiva, anaemia
  Anaemia: If the lower lid is everted, the colour of the mucous membrane can be seen. If these are pale, the haemoglobin is usually $< 9\,g\,dl^{-1}$.
- eyelids: white/yellow deposit, *xanthelasma* (Xanthelasma may be familial or related to hypercholesteremia.)
- puffy eyelids
  general oedema, e.g. *nephrotic syndrome*
  thyroid eye disease, hyper or hypo
  myxoedema
- red eye
  iritis (*uveitis* – anterior/posterior. This must be considered a medical emergency.)
  conjunctivitis
  scleritis or *episcleritis*
  acute *glaucoma* (This must be considered a medical emergency.)
- white line around cornea, *arcus senilis*
  common and of little significance in the elderly
  suggests *hyperlipidaemia* in younger patients
- white-band keratopathy-hypercalcaemia
  sarcoid

parathyroid tumour or *hyperplasia*
lung oat-cell tumour
bone secondaries
vitamin D excess intake

Hypercalcaemia may give a horizontal band across exposed medial and lateral parts of cornea.

- white growth of bulbar conjunctival tissue
Pterygium (Usually occurs from the nasal side towards the centre of the cornea. It may interfere with vision if it covers the pupil.) (Solomer and Bowling 2018)

2.7 Examine the Fundi

This is often done as part of the neurological system (see Chapter 11) when examining the cranial nerves. It is placed here as features are also covered in the general examination.

- Use ophthalmoscope
    - The patient should be sitting. Remove spectacles from yourself and the patient.
    - Begin by setting the lens dioptre dial at 0 if you do not use spectacles. If you are myopic, you should start with the 'minus' lenses. Set the lens dioptre at −4 to begin, which is indicated as a red number. If you are hyperopic you should use the 'plus' lenses, which are indicated by black numbers. Keep your index finger on the dial to permit easy focusing. Hold the ophthalmoscope about 30 cm from the patient, shine the light into the patient's pupil, identify the red reflex (from the retina), and approach the patient at an angle of 15°.

Approach on the same horizontal plane as the equator of the patient's eye. This will bring you straight to the patient's optic disc. After observing the disc examine the peripheral retina fully by following the blood vessels to and back from the four main quadrants.

  - Hold the ophthalmoscope in your right hand in front of your right eye to examine the patient's right eye and your left eye to examine the patient's left eye. Try to hold your breath when using the ophthalmoscope. Do not breathe into the patient's face.
  - If the patient's pupils are small, dilate with 1% tropicamide, 1 drop per eye. Works in 15–20 minutes and lasts two to four hours. Warn the patient that vision will be blurred for approximately four hours. Do **not** dilate if neurological observation of pupils is needed.
  - The patient should be told not to drive, if pupils have been dilated, for at least four to six hours (Cox 2010).

- Look at optic disc
  - normally pink rim with white 'cup' below surface of disc
  - *optic atrophy*
    - disc pale: rim no longer pink
      multiple sclerosis
      after optic neuritis
      optic nerve compression, e.g. *tumour*
  - papilloedema
    - disc pink, indistinct margin
    - cup disappears
    - dilated retinal veins
      increased cerebral pressure, e.g. *tumour*
      accelerated hypertension
      optic neuritis, acute stage

  - glaucoma – enlarged cup, diminished rim
  - new vessels – new fronds of vessels coming forwards from discischaemic diabetic retinopathy
- Look at arteries
  - arteries narrowed in hypertension, with increased light reflex along top of vessel
    Hypertension grading:
    1. narrow arteries
    2. 'nipping' (narrowing of veins by arteries)
    3. flame-shaped haemorrhages (e.g. hypertension) and cotton-wool spots (e.g. hyperlipidemia; atherosclerosis)
    4. papilloedema.
  - occlusion artery – pale retina
    occlusion vein – haemorrhages (Kanski 2009; Solomer and Bowling 2018)
- Look at retina
  - hard exudates (shiny, yellow circumscribed patches of lipid)
    diabetes
  - cotton-wool spots (soft, fluffy white patches)
    microinfarcts causing local swelling of nerve fibres
      diabetes
      hypertension
      vasculitis
      human immunodeficiency virus (HIV)
  - small, red dots
    microaneurysms – retinal capillary expansion adjacent to capillary closure
      diabetes
  - haemorrhages
    - round 'blots': haemorrhages deep in retina larger than microaneurysms
      diabetes

    - flame-shaped: superficial haemorrhages along nerve fibres
      hypertension
      gross anaemia
      hyperviscosity
      bleeding tendency
    - Roth's spots (white-centred haemorrhages)
      microembolic disorder
      subacute bacterial endocarditis
  - pigmentation
    widespread
      retinitis pigmentosa
    localised
      choroiditis (clumping of pigment into patches)
      drug toxicity, e.g. chloroquine
    tigroid or tabby fundus: normal variant in choroid beneath retina
  - peripheral new vessels
    ischaemic *diabetic retinopathy*
    retinal *vein occlusion*
  - medullated nerve fibres – normal variant, areas of white nerves radiating from optic disc (see Chapter 11) (Kanski 2009; Solomer and Bowling 2018)

2.8 Examine for Palpable Lymph Nodes

- In the neck:
  - above clavicle (posterior triangle)
  - medial to sternomastoid area (anterior triangle)
  - submandibular (can palpate submandibular gland)
  - occipital

These glands are best felt by sitting the patient up and examining from behind. A left supraclavicular node can occur from the spread of a gastrointestinal malignancy (Virchow's node).

- In the axillae:
  - abduct arm, insert your hand along lateral side of axilla, and adduct arm, thus placing your fingertips in the apex of the axilla. Palpate gently
- In the epitrochlear region:
  - medial to and above elbow
- In the groins:
  - over inguinal ligament
- In the abdomen:
  - usually very difficult to feel; some claim to have felt para-aortic nodes

    Axillae often have soft, fleshy lymph nodes.
    Groins often have small, shotty nodes.
    Generalised large, rubbery nodes suggest *lymphoma*.
    Localised hard nodes suggest *cancer.*
    Tender nodes suggest *infection*.
- If many nodes are palpable – examine spleen and look for anaemia. *Lymphoma or leukaemia*? (Cox 2010; Talley and O'Connor 2006, 2014).

2.9 Lumps

- If there is an unusual lump, inspect first and palpate later:
  - site
  - size (measure in centimetres)
  - shape
  - surface, edge
  - surroundings
  - fixed or mobile

  - consistency, e.g. cystic or solid, soft or hard, fluctuance
  - tender
  - pulsatile
  - auscultation, e.g. thyroid 'hum' from increased vascularity
  - transillumination

  A *cancer* is usually hard, nontender, irregular, fixed to neighbouring tissues, and possibly ulcerating skin.

  A *cyst* may have:

    - fluctuance: pressure across cyst will cause it to bulge in another plane
    - transillumination: a light can be seen through it (usually only if room is darkened).

- Look at neighbouring lymph nodes. May find:
  - spread from cancer
  - inflamed lymph nodes from infection (Swartz 2014)

2.10 Heart

2.10.1 Routine Examination

For the full examination refer to Chapter 4, Examination of the Cardiovascular System.

- Inspect precordium
  - observe point of maximum impulse (usually fifth intercostal space [ICS] in an adult)
  - look for heaves
- Palpate precordium
  - heaves or thrusts
  - thrills (palpable murmurs/vibrations)

- Percuss precordium
    - heart will enlarge in congestive heart failure and cardiomegaly
    - apex may shift laterally to the left and be located in the sixth ICS
- Auscultate: S_1, S_2 (? S_3, S_4, clicks, snaps, or murmurs)
    - rate
    - rhythm (regular, regular – irregular)
- Assess jugular venous distension/jugular venous pressure (JVD/JVP) (Cox 2010)

2.11 Breasts

If you are a male, arrange for a female chaperone, particularly when the patient is a young adult, shy, or nervous (Cox 2010).

2.11.1 Routine Examination

- Examine the female breasts when you examine the precordium.
- Inspect for asymmetry, obvious lumps, inverted nipples, skin changes.
- Palpate each quadrant of both breasts with the flat of the hand (fingers together, nearly extended with gentle pressure exerted from metacarpophalangeal joints, avoiding pressure on the nipple).
- If there are any possible lumps, proceed to a more complete examination.

2.11.2 Full Breast Examination

When patient has a symptom or a lump has been found:

- Inspect
    - With the patient sitting up ask the patient to raise her hands above her head, put hands on hips, rotate shoulders forwards, and then with

hands on hips to lean forwards (so that you can examine under the breast). Look anteriorly and laterally.

- Inspect for asymmetry or obvious lumps
    - differing size or shape of breasts
    - nipples – symmetry
    - rashes, redness (abscess)

    Breast cancer is suggested by:
        - asymmetry
        - skin tethering or puckering
        - *peau d'orange* (oedema of skin)
        - nipple deviated or inverted.

- Palpate
    - Patient lying flat on one pillow with one arm under her head and other at her side (right arm under head to examine right breast and left arm under head to examine left breast)
    - Examine each breast with flat of hand, each quadrant in turn (ensure that you examine well below each breast and into the tail of Spence)
    - Examine bimanually if large
    - Examine any lump as described in the General Inspection on skin and lymph nodes (this chapter)
        - is lump attached to skin or muscles?
        - examine lymph nodes (axilla, infraclavicular, and supraclavicular)
        - feel liver (Ball et al. 2014a; Cox 2010; Seidel et al. 2006, 2010).

2.12 Respiratory

2.12.1 Routine Examination

For the full examination refer to Chapter 5, Examination of the Respiratory System.

- Inspect:
  - symmetry (? flail, tracheal deviation)
  - scars/lesions
  - respiratory rate
  - ? nasal flaring
- Palpate:
  - thoracic integrity
  - lumps/bumps
  - crepitations
  - fremitus
- Percuss:
  - anteriorly
  - posteriorly
  - laterally
  - ? dullness on percussion (consolidation or tumour)
- Auscultate:
  - tracheobronchial sounds
  - bronchovesicular sounds
  - vesicular sounds
  - ? adventitious sounds (Ball et al. 2014a; Cox 2010; Dains et al. 2015; Epstein et al. 2008; Jarvis 2015).

2.13 Thyroid

- Inspect: then give the patient a glass of water and ask them to swallow. Is there a lump? Does it move upwards on swallowing?
- Palpate bimanually: stand behind the patient and palpate with fingers of both hands. Is the thyroid of normal size, shape, and texture? (Avoid the throttling position when examining behind the patient as this may frighten the patient.)

- If a lump is felt:
  - is thyroid multinodular?
  - does lump feel cystic?

    The thyroid is normally soft. If there is a goitre (swelling of thyroid), assess if the swelling is:
    - localised, e.g. *thyroid cyst*, *adenoma*, or *carcinoma*
    - generalised, e.g. *autoimmune thyroiditis, thyrotoxicosis*
    - multinodular.

    A swelling does not mean the gland is under- or overactive. In many cases the patient may be euthyroid. The thyroid becomes slightly enlarged in pregnancy.
- Ask patient to swallow – does thyroid rise normally?
- Is thyroid fixed?
- Can you get below the lump? If not, percuss over upper sternum for retrosternal extension
- Are there cervical lymph nodes?
- If possibility of patient being thyrotoxic, look for:
  - warm hands
  - perspiration
  - tremor
  - tachycardia, sinus rhythm, or atrial fibrillation
  - wide, palpable fissure or lid lag
  - thyroid 'hum' – bruit (on auscultation)

    Endocrine exophthalmos (may be associated with thyrotoxicosis):
    - conjunctival oedema: *chemosis* (seen by gentle pressure on lower lid, pushing up a fold of conjunctiva when oedema is present)
    - proptosis: eye pushed forwards (look from above down on eyes)
    - deficient upwards gaze and convergence

    - diplopia
    - papilloedema.
- If possibility of patient being *hypothyroid*, look for:
    - dry hair and skin
    - xanthelasma
    - puffy face
    - croaky voice
    - delayed relaxation of supinator or ankle jerks (Ball et al. 2014a; Cox 2010; Dains et al. 2015; Epstein et al. 2008; Jarvis 2015).

2.14 Other Endocrine Diseases

2.14.1 Acromegaly

- enlarged soft tissue of hands, feet, face
- coarse features; thick, greasy skin; large tongue (and other organs, e.g. thyroid)
- bitemporal hemianopia (from tumour pressing on optic chiasma)

2.14.2 Hypopituitarism

- no skin pigmentation
- thin skin
- decreased secondary sexual hair or delayed puberty
- short stature (and on X-ray, delayed fusion of epiphyses)
- bitemporal hemianopia if pituitary tumour

2.14.3 Addison's Disease

- increased skin pigmentation, including nonexposed areas, e.g. buccal pigmentation
- postural hypotension
- if female, decreased body hair

2.14.4 Cushing's Syndrome

- truncal obesity; round, red face with hirsutism
- thin skin and bruising, pink striae, hypertension
- proximal muscle weakness

2.14.5 Diabetes

Diabetic complications include:

- skin lesions
  Necrobiosis lipoidica – ischaemia in skin, usually on shins, leading to fatty replacement of dermis, covered by thin skin.
- ischaemic legs
  - diminished foot pulses
  - skin shiny blue, white, or black
  - no hairs, thick nails
  - ulcers
- peripheral neuropathy
  - absent leg reflexes
  - diminished sensation
  - thick skin over unusual pressure points from dropped arch
- autonomic neuropathy
  - dry skin
- mononeuropathy
  - lateral popliteal nerve – footdrop
  - III or VI – diplopia
  - asymmetrical muscle-wasting of the upper leg
- retinopathy (Ball et al. 2014a; Cox 2010; Dains et al. 2015; Epstein et al. 2008; Jarvis 2015).

2.15 Abdomen

For palpation and percussion, the abdomen is divided into nine imaginary quadrants (with components identified as right hypochondrial, epigastric, left hypochondrial, umbilical, left lumbar, left iliac (or hypogastric), suprapubic (or hypogastric), right hypogastric, right lumbar and umbilical) Figure 2.1.

For auscultation the abdomen is divided into four imaginary quadrants (with components identified as right upper quadrant, left upper quadrant, left lower quadrant and right lower quadrant [Table 2.1]).

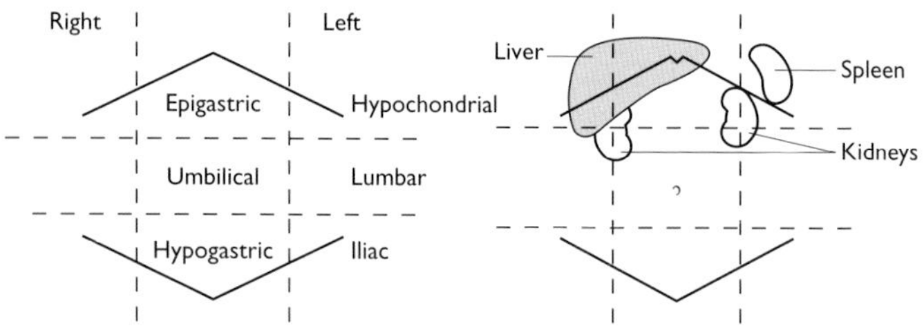

Figure 2.1 Nine abdominal quadrants and location of organs in epigastric, hypochondrial, and lumbar regions. Source: Cox 2010. Reproduced with permission from John Wiley and Sons.

Table 2.1 Distribution of components in the four imaginary quadrants of the abdomen.

Right upper quadrant (RUQ)	**Left upper quadrant (LUQ)**
Liver	Stomach
Gall bladder	Spleen
Head of pancreas	Body of pancreas
Right kidney	Left kidney
Large intestine	Large intestine
Small intestine	Small intestine
Right lower quadrant (RLQ)	**Left lower quadrant (LLQ)**
Appendix	
Right ovary	Left ovary
Large intestine	Large intestine
Small intestine	Small intestine
	Uterus
	Bladder

2.15.1 Routine Examination

Inspect:
  - symmetry (? concave or convex)
  - scars/lesions (? evidence of liver disease)
- Auscultate:
  - four quadrants
- Palpate:
  - nine quadrants (light and deep palpation)
  - lumps/bumps (? presence of tumour)
- Percuss:
  - nine quadrants
  - tympani
  - ? central dullness and lateral tympani (ovarian tumour)
  - ? central tympani and lateral dullness (ascites – assess for shifting dullness)
  - consider rectal/vaginal examination (Ball et al. 2014a; Cox 2010; Dains et al. 2015; Epstein et al. 2008; Japp and Robertson 2013; Jarvis 2008, 2015; Rhoads and Paterson 2013; Rundio and Lorman 2017).

2.16 Musculoskeletal

Normally you would examine the joints briefly when examining neighbouring systems. If a patient specifically complains of joint symptoms or an abnormal posture or joint is noted, a more detailed examination is needed (Cox 2010).

2.16.1 General Habitus

- Note the following:
  - is the patient unduly tall or short? (measure height and span)
  - are all limbs, spine, and skull of normal size and shape?

    - normal person:
      height = span
      crown to pubis = pubis to heel
    - long limbs:
      Marfan's syndrome
      eunuchoid during growth
    - *collapsed vertebrae*:
      span > height
      pubis to heel > crown to pubis
- is the posture normal?
- curvature of the spine:
  kyphosis
  lordosis
  scoliosis
  gibbus
- is the gait normal?
  Observing the patient walking is a vital part of examination of the locomotor system and neurological system.

  Painful gait, transferring weight quickly off a painful limb, bobbing up and down – an abnormal rhythm of gait.

  Painless abnormal gait may be from:

  short leg (bobs up and down with equal-length steps)

  stiff joint (lifts pelvis to prevent foot dragging on ground)

  weak ankle (high stepping gait to avoid toes catching on ground)

  weak knee (locks knee straight before putting foot on the ground)

  weak hip (sways sideways using trunk muscles to lift pelvis and to swing leg through)

  uncoordinated gait (arms are swung as counterbalances)

  hysterical or malingering causes.

Look for abnormal wear on shoes.

2.16.2 Inspection

Inspect the joints before you touch them.

- Look at:
  - skin
    redness – inflammation
    scars – old injury
    bruising – recent injury
  - soft tissues
    muscle wasting – old injury
    swelling – injury/inflammation
  - bones
    deformity – compare with other side
    varus: bent out from midline (bowleg)
    valgus: bent in towards midline
- Assess whether an isolated joint is affected, or if there is polyarthritis.
- If there is polyarthritis, note if it is symmetrical or asymmetrical.
- Compare any abnormal findings with the other side.

Arthritis – swollen, hot, tender, painful joint.

Arthropathy – swollen but not hot and tender.

Arthralgia – painful, e.g. *on movement, without being swollen.*

Swelling may also be due to an effusion, thickening of the periarticular tissues, enlargement of the ends of bones (e.g. *pulmonary osteopathy*), or complete disorganisation of the joint without pain (*Charcot's joint*).

2.16.3 Palpation

- Before you touch any joint ask the patient to tell you if it is painful.
- Feel for:
  - warmth
  - tenderness

    - watch patient's face for signs of discomfort
    - locate signs of tenderness – soft tissue or bone
  - swelling or displacement
  - fluctuation (effusion)

    An inflamed joint is usually generally tender. Localised tenderness may be mechanical in origin, e.g. ligament tear. Joint effusion may occur with an arthritis or local injury.

2.16.4 Movement

Test the range of movement (ROM) of the joint both actively and passively. This must be done gently.

- Active – how far can the patient move the joint through its range?

  Do not seize limb and move it until patient complains.
- Passive – if range is limited, can you further increase the range of movement?

  Abduction: movement away from central axis.

  Adduction: movement toward central axis.

  is the passive range of movement similar to the active range?

  Limitation of the range of movement of a joint may be due to pain, muscle spasms, contracture, inflammation or thickening of the capsules or periarticular structures, effusions into the joint space, bony or cartilaginous outgrowths, or painful conditions not connected with the joint.
- Resisted movement – ask patient to bend joint whilst you resist movement. How much force can be developed?
- Hold your hand round the joint whilst it is moving. A grating or creaking sensation (*crepitus*) may be felt.

  Crepitus is usually associated with *osteoarthritis*.

2.16.5 Summary of Signs of Common Illnesses

2.16.5.1 *Osteoarthritis*

- 'wear and tear' of a specific joint – usually large joints
- common in elderly or after trauma to joint
- often involves joints of the lower limbs and is asymmetrical
- often in the lumbar or cervical spine
- aches after use, with deep, boring pain at night
- Heberden's nodes – osteophytes on terminal interphalangeal joints

2.16.5.2 *Rheumatoid Arthritis*

Characteristically:

- a polyarthritis
- symmetrical, inflamed if active
- involves proximal interphalangeal and metacarpophalangeal joints of hands with ulnar deviation of fingers
- involves any large joint
- muscle wasting from disuse atrophy
- rheumatoid nodules on extensor surface of elbows
- may include other signs, e.g. with splenomegaly it is *Felty's syndrome*

2.16.5.3 *Gout*

Characteristically:

- asymmetrical
- inflamed first metatarsophalangeal joint (big toe) – *podagra*

- involves any joint in hand, often with tophus – hard round lump of urate by joint
- tophi on ears

2.16.5.4 Psoriasis

- particularly involves terminal interphalangeal joints, hips, and knees
- often with pitted nails of psoriasis as well as skin lesions

2.16.5.5 Ankylosing Spondylitis

- painful, stiff spine
- later fixed in flexed position
- hips and other joints can be involved (Ball et al. 2014a; Cox 2010; Dains et al. 2012, 2015; Epstein et al. 2008; Japp and Robertson 2013; Jarvis 2008, 2015; Rhoads and Paterson 2013; Rundio and Lorman 2017).

References

Ball, J., Dains, J., Flynn, J. et al. (2014a). *Seidel's Guide to Physical Examination*, 8e. St. Louis: Mosby.

Ball, J., Dains, J., Flynn, J. et al. (2014b). *Student Laboratory Manual to Accompany Seidel's Guide to Physical Examination*, 8e. St. Louis: Mosby.

Barkauskas, V., Baumann, L., and Darling-Fisher, C. (2002). *Health and Physical Assessment*, 3e. London: Mosby.

Bickley, L. and Szilagyi, P. (2007). *Bates' Guide to Physical Examination and History Taking*, 7e. Philadelphia: Lippincott.

Bickley, L. and Szilagyi, P. (2013). *Bates' Guide to Physical Examination and History Taking*, 11e. New York: Wolters Kluwer/Lippincott Williams & Wilkins.

Collins-Bride, G. and Saxe, J. (2013). *Clinical Guidelines for Advanced Practice Nursing – An Interdisciplinary Approach*, 2e. Burlington, MA: Jones and Bartlett Learning.

Coulehan, J. (2006). *The Medical Interview: Mastering Skills for Clinical Practice*, 5e. Philadelphia: F. A. David Company.

Cox, C. (2010). *Physical Assessment for Nurses*, 2e. Oxford: Wiley Blackwell.

Dains, J., Baumann, L., and Scheibel, P. (2012). *Advanced Health Assessment and Clinical Diagnosis in Primary Care*, 4e. St. Louis: Elsevier.

Dains, J., Baumann, L., and Scheibel, P. (2015). *Advanced Health Assessment and Clinical Diagnosis in Primary Care*, 5e. St. Louis: Mosby.

Epstein, O., Perkin, G., de Bono, D., and Cookson, J. (2008). *Clinical Examination*, 4e. London: Mosby.

Hatton, C. and Blackwood, R. (2003). *Lecture Notes on Clinical Skills*, 4e. Oxford: Blackwell Science.

Japp, A. and Robertson, C. (2013). *Macleod's Clinical Diagnosis*. Edinburgh: Churchill Livingstone, Elsevier.

Jarvis, C. (2008). *Physical Examination and Health Assessment*, 5e. St. Louis: Saunders.

Jarvis, C. (2015). *Physical Examination and Health Assessment*, 7e. Edinburgh: Elsevier.

Kanski, J. (2009). *Clinical Ophthamology, a Synopsis*, 2e. London: Butterworth Heinemann Elsevier.

Lack, V. (2012). Consultation skills. In: *Advanced Practice in Healthcare* (ed. C. Cox, M. Hill and V. Lack), 39–56. London: Routledge.

Rhoads, J. and Paterson, S. (2013). *Advanced Health Assessment and Diagnostic Reasoning*, 2e. Burlington: Jones and Bartlett.

Rundio, A. and Lorman, W. (2017). *Lippincott Certification Review: Family Nurse Practitioner & Adult-Gerontology Nurse Practitioner.* London: Wolters Kluwer.

Seidel, H., Ball, J., Dains, J., and Benedict, G. (2006). *Mosby's Physical Examination Handbook*. St. Louis: Mosby.

Seidel, H., Ball, J., Dains, J., and Benedict, G. (2010). *Mosby's Physical Examination Handbook*, 7e. St. Louis: Mosby-Year Book.

Solomer, J. and Bowling, B. (2018). *Kanski's Clinical Ophthalmology, a Systematic Approach*. London: Elsevier.

Swartz, M. (2006). *Physical Diagnosis, History and Examination*, 5e. London: W. B. Saunders.

Swartz, M. (2014). *Physical Diagnosis: History and Examination*, With Student Consult Online Access, 7e. London: Elsevier.

Talley, N. and O'Connor, S. (2006). *Clinical Examination: A Systematic Guide to Physical Diagnosis*, 5e. London: Churchill Livingstone.

Talley, N. and O'Connor, S. (2014). *Clinical Examination: A Systematic Guide to Physical Diagnosis*, 7e. London: Churchill Livingstone, Elsevier.

3 Basic Examination, Notes, and Diagnostic Principles

Carol Lynn Cox[1,2]
[1] *School of Health Sciences, City, University of London, London, UK*
[2] *Health and Hope Clinics, Pensacola, FL, USA*

3.1 Basic Examination

3.1.1 Introduction

In practice, you cannot attempt to elicit every single physical sign for each system. Your examination will be guided by the patient's chief complaint and presenting history. Basic signs should be sought on every examination, and if there is any hint of abnormality, additional physical signs can be elicited to confirm your suspicion (Bickley and Szilagyi 2007, 2013; Collins-Bride and Saxe 2013; Dains et al. 2012, 2015; Japp and Robertson 2013; Jarvis 2015; Seidel et al. 2006, 2010; Swartz 2006, 2014).

The basic examination of systems is listed below:

Review of Systems (ROS). At the initial stage of the examination ensure that you fully review systems from the patient's perspective. These are subjective views presented by the patient. This will guide your basic examination. For example, Peripheral Vascular System (PVS) 'Patient notes bruising on legs and arms.' Follow the ROS with your General Examination.

Pocket Guide to Physical Assessment, First Edition. Edited by Carol Lynn Cox.

The order of examining each system is delineated below:

- General examination
    - general appearance
    - is the patient well or ill?
    - look at temperature chart or take patient's temperature
    - any obvious abnormality?
    - mental health state, mood, behaviour
- General and cardiovascular system
    - observation – dyspnoea, distress
    - O_2 saturation
    - blood pressure
    - hands
    - temperature
    - nails, e.g. clubbing, leukonychia, koilonychias, palmar erythema
    - pulse – rate, rhythm, character
    - axillae – lymph nodes
    - neck – lymph nodes
    - face and eyes – anaemia, jaundice
    - tongue and mucus membranes – central cyanosis
    - jugular venous pulse (JVP)/jugular venous distension (JVD) – height and v wave
    - apex beat/point of maximal impulse (PMI) – position and character
    - parasternal – heave or thrills
    - stethoscope
        - heart sounds (S_1 and S_2), added sounds (clicks or snaps), splits (? physiological split), murmurs
        - listen in all five areas with stethoscope using the bell and diaphragm
        - lay patient on left side, with the bell of stethoscope listen for mitral stenosis (MS)

        - sit patient up, have them lean forwards and breathe out, with bell of stethoscope listen for aortic incompetence (AI)
- Respiratory system
    - observation (scars, lesions, ecchymoses)
    - trachea – position
    - front of chest
        - movement (respiratory excursion; flail)
        - palpate (lumps, crepitus, fremitus)
        - percuss – compare sides
        - auscultate – compare sides
    - back of chest
        - movement (respiratory excursion)
        - palpate (lumps, crepitus, fremitus)
        - percuss – particularly level of bases (diaphragmatic excursion); compare sides
        - auscultate – compare sides
    - examine sputum
- Examine spine (? lordosis, kyphosis, scoliosis, gibbus)
- Abdomen
    - lay patient flat (knees bent to relax abdomen)
    - look at abdomen – ask if pain or tenderness
    - auscultate in all four quadrants (include aortic, iliac and femoral arteries/? bruits)
    - palpate abdomen gently
        - generally all over? masses
        - liver – then percuss
        - spleen – then percuss
        - kidneys
        - (shifting dullness – ascites if indicated)
    - feel femoral pulses and inguinal lymph nodes
    - hernia
    - males – genitals
    - per rectum (PR; only if given permission) – usually at end of examination
    - per vaginam (PV; only if given permission) – usually at end of examination

- Legs
  - observation
  - arterial pulses (joints if indicated)
  - neurology

– reflexes	– knees	tone	only if indicated
	– ankles	power	
	– plantar responses	coordination	
– sensation	– pinprick	position	
	– vibration	cotton-wool	
		temperature	

- Arms
  - posture: outstretched hands, eyes closed, rapid finger movements
  - finger–nose coordination

– reflexes	– triceps	tone	only if indicated
	– biceps	power	
	– supinator		
		vibration	
– sensation	– pinprick	position	
		cotton-wool	
		temperature	

- Cranial nerves
  - I (if indicated)
  - II: eyes
    - reading print/acuity
    - fields

  - pupils – torch and accommodation
  - ophthalmoscope – sclera, cornea, anterior chamber, and posterior fundi
- III, IV, VI: eye movements (Extraocular Muscles [EOM])
  - 'Do you see double?'
  - note nystagmus
- V, VII
  - open mouth
  - grit teeth – feel masseters
  - sensation – cotton-wool
  - (corneal reflex – if indicated)
  - (taste – if indicated)
- VIII: hearing
  - watch at each ear
  - (Rinne, Weber tests if indicated)
- IX, X: fauces movement
- XI: shrug shoulders
- XII: put out tongue

- Walk – look at gait
- Hernia and varicose veins

3.2 Example of Notes

You may find the SOAPIER (Subjective, Objective, Assessment, Plan, Implementation, Evaluation, Review) format or POMR (Problem Oriented Medical Record) useful in documenting your findings (Clark 1999; Jarvis 2015; Swartz 2006, 2014).

Patient's name: Age: Occupation:

Date of admission:

Complains of (chief complaint):

- list, in patient's words

History of present illness:

- detailed description of each symptom (even if appears irrelevant) (Note language barriers that may have an impact on documentation.)
- last well
- chronological order, with both actual date of onset, and time previous to admission
- (may include history from informant – in which case, state this is so)
- then detail other questions which seem relevant to possible differential diagnoses
- then **functional enquiry**, 'check' system for other symptoms
- (minimal statement in notes – weight, appetite, digestion, bowels, micturition, menstruation, if appropriate)

Past history:

- chronological order

Family history:

- include genogram

Personal and social history:

- must include details of home circumstances, dependents, patient's occupation
- effect of illness on life and its relevance to foreseeable discharge of patient
- smoking, alcohol, drug misuse, medications

Medications:

- list all medications the patient is presently taking

Allergies:

Physical examination:

- general appearance
- then record findings according to systems

Minimal statement:

Healthy, well-nourished woman (or man)

Afebrile, not anaemic, icteric, or cyanosed

No enlargement of lymph nodes

No clubbing

Breasts/chest and thyroid normal

Patient's name:	**Age:** **Occupation:**
Cerebrovascular system (CVS):	Blood pressure, pulse rate, and rhythm
	JVP not raised
	Apex position
	Heart sounds 1 and 2, no murmurs
Respiratory system:	Cyanosis (present/absent)
	O_2 saturation
	Chest and movements normal
	Fremitus normal
	Percussion note normal
	Breath sounds bilateral/vesicular
	No other (adventitious) sounds
Abdominal system:	Tongue and mucus membranes normal
	Abdomen normal, no tenderness
	Liver, spleen, kidneys, bladder impalpable
	No masses felt
	Hernial orifices normal
	Rectal examination normal
	Vaginal examination not performed
	Testes normal
Central nervous system (CNS):	Alert and intelligent
	Pupils equal, regular, react equally to light and accommodation (PERRLA)
	Fundi normal
	Normal eye movements
	Other cranial nerves normal
	Limbs normal
	Knee jerks + +
	Ankle jerks + +
	Plantar reflexes ↓ ↓
	Touch and vibration normal
	Spine and joints normal
	Gait normal
	Pulses (including dorsalis pedis, posterior tibial, and popliteal) palpable

3.2.1 Summary

Write a few sentences only:

- salient positive features of history and examination
- relevant negative information
- home circumstances
- patient's mental state
    - understanding of illness
    - specific concerns

3.3 Problem List and Diagnoses

After your history and examination, make a list of:

- the diagnoses you have been able to make
- problems or abnormal findings which need explaining.

For example:

- symptoms or signs
- anxiety
- poor social background
- laboratory results
- drug sensitivities

It is best to separate the current problems of actual or potential clinical significance requiring treatment or follow-up from the inactive problems. An example is:

Active problems	**Date**
1. Unexplained episodes of fainting	one week
2. Angina	since 2012
3. Hypertension – blood pressure 190/100 mmHg	2012

Active problems	Date
4. Chronic renal failure – plasma creatinine 200 μmol l^{-1}	August 2014
5. Widower, unemployed, lives on own	
6. Anxious about possibility of being injured in a fall	
7. Smokes 40 cigarettes per day	

Inactive problems	Date
1. Thyrotoxicosis treated by partial thyroidectomy	2000
2. ACE inhibitor-induced cough	2011

When you initially begin examining patients you will have difficulty knowing which problems to put down separately and which can be covered under one diagnosis and a single entry. It is therefore advisable to rewrite the problem list if a problem resolves or can be explained by a diagnosis. When you are more experienced, it will be appropriate to fill out the problems on a complete problem list at the front of the notes. Use medical diagnoses in the medical notes.

Active problems	Date	Inactive problems	Date
Include symptoms, signs, unexplained abnormal investigations, social and psychiatric problems		Include major past illness, operation, or hypersensitivities; do not include problems requiring active care	

From the problem list, you should be able to make:

- differential diagnoses, including that which you think is most likely. Remember:
- common diseases occur commonly
- an unusual manifestation of a common disease is more likely than an uncommon disease

- do not necessarily be put off by some aspect which does not fit
- possible diagnostic investigations you feel are appropriate
- management and therapy you think are appropriate
- prognostic implications

3.3.1 Diagnoses

The diagnostic terms which are used often relate to different levels of understanding:

Disordered function	Immobile painful joint	Breathlessness	Angina
	↑	↑	↑
Structural lesion	Osteoarthritis	Anaemia	Narrow coronary artery
	↑	↑	↑
Pathology	Iron-deposition fibrosis (haemochromatosis)	Iron deficiency	Aortitis
	↑	↑	↑
Aetiology	Inherited disorder of iron metabolism – homozygous for C282Y with A-H	Bleeding duodenal ulcer	*Treponema pallidum* (syphilis)

Different problems require diagnoses at different levels, which may change as further information becomes available. Thus, a patient initially may be diagnosed as *pyrexia of unknown origin*. After a plain X-ray of the abdomen, the patient may be found to have a *renal mass* which on a computed tomography (CT) scan becomes *perinephric abscess*, which from blood cultures is found to be *Staphylococcus aureus* infection. For a complete diagnosis all aspects should be known, but often this is not possible (Bickley and Szilagyi 2013; Collins-Bride and Saxe 2013; Dains et al. 2012, 2015; Japp and Robertson 2013; Jarvis 2015; Seidel et al. 2006, 2010; Swartz 2006, 2014).

Note that many terms are used as a diagnosis but, in fact, cover considerable ignorance, e.g. *diabetes mellitus* (originally 'sweet-tasting urine', but now also diagnosed by high plasma glucose) is no more than a descriptive term of disordered function. *Sarcoid* relates to a pattern of symptoms and a pathology of noncaseating granulomata, of which the aetiology is unknown.

3.3.2 Progress Notes

The electronic patient record has become the norm in most healthcare environments. In the general practice surgery, clinic, or primary care facility, full progress notes should give a complete picture of:

- how the diagnosis was established
- how the patient was treated
- the evolution of the illness
- any complications that occurred

These notes are as important as the account of the original examination. In acute cases, record daily changes in signs and symptoms. In chronic cases, the relevant systems should be reexamined at least once a week and the findings recorded.

It is useful to separate different aspects of the illness:

- symptoms
- signs
- laboratory investigations
- general assessment, e.g. apparent response to therapy
- further plans, which would include educating the patient and his family about the illness

Objective findings such as alterations in weight, improvement in colour, pulse, character of respirations, or fluid intake and output are more valuable than purely subjective statements such as 'General improvement from previous examination'.

When appropriate, daily blood pressure readings or analyses of the urine should be recorded.

An account of all procedures such as aspirations of chest should be included.

Specifically record:

- the findings and comments of the physician, surgeon, or advanced registered nurse practitioner (ARNP) managing the case
- results of a case conference
- an opinion from another department

3.3.3 Serial Investigations

The results of these should be collected together in a table on a special sheet. When any large series of investigations is made, e.g. serial blood counts, erythrocyte sedimentation rates, or multiple biochemical analyses, the results can also be expressed by a graph.

3.3.4 Operation Notes

If you are working in a team where patients are undergoing surgical treatment, you may be required to write an operation note following surgery. An operation note must be written immediately after the operation. Do not trust your memory for any length of time as several similar problems may be operated on at one session. Even if you are distracted by an emergency, the notes must be written up the same day as the operation. These notes should contain definite statements on the following facts:

- name of surgeon performing the operation and the surgical assistant
- name of anaesthetist and anaesthetic used
- type and dimension of incision used
- pathological condition found and mention of anatomical variations
- operative procedures carried out
- method of repair of wound and suture materials used
- whether drainage used, material used, and whether sutured to wound
- type of dressing used.

3.3.5 Postoperative Notes

Within the first two days after an operation note:

- the general condition of the patient
- any complication or troublesome symptom, e.g. pain, haemorrhage, vomiting, distension, etc.
- any treatment.

3.3.6 Discharge Note from Hospital

A full statement of the patient's condition on discharge should be written:

- final diagnosis
- active problems
- medication and other therapies
- plan
- what the patient has been told: education (patient teaching) given on medications, diagnosis, and other pertinent information (e.g. blood pressure monitoring)
- specific follow-up points, e.g. persistent depressive disorder

- where the patient has gone, and what help is available
- when the patient is next being seen
- an estimate of the prognosis.

References

Bickley, L. and Szilagyi, P. (2007). *Bates' Guide to Physical Examination and History Taking*, 9e. Philadelphia: Lippincott.

Bickley, L. and Szilagyi, P. (2013). *Bates' Guide to Physical Examination and History Taking*, 11e. New York: Wolters Kluwer/Lippincott Williams & Wilkins.

Clark, C. (1999). Taking a history. In: *Nurse Practitioners, Clinical Skills and Professional Issues* (ed. M. Walsh, A. Crumbie and S. Reveley), 12–23. Oxford: Butterworth Heinemann.

Collins-Bride, G. and Saxe, J. (2013). *Clinical Guidelines for Advanced Practice Nursing – An Interdisciplinary Approach*, 2e. Burlington, MA: Jones and Bartlett Learning.

Dains, J., Baumann, L., and Scheibel, P. (2012). *Advanced Health Assessment and Clinical Diagnosis in Primary Care*, 4e. St. Louis: Elsevier.

Dains, J., Baumann, L., and Scheibel, P. (2015). *Advanced Health Assessment and Clinical Diagnosis in Primary Care*, 5e. St. Louis: Mosby.

Japp, A. and Robertson, C. (2013). *Macleod's Clinical Diagnosis*. Edinburgh: Churchill Livingstone, Elsevier.

Jarvis, C. (2015). *Physical Examination and Health Assessment*, 7e. Edinburgh: Elsevier.

Seidel, H., Ball, J., Dains, J., and Benedict, G. (2006). *Mosby's Physical Examination Handbook*. St. Louis: Mosby.

Seidel, H., Ball, J., Dains, J., and Benedict, G. (2010). *Mosby's Physical Examination Handbook*, 7e. St. Louis: Mosby-Year Book.

Swartz, M. (2006). *Physical Diagnosis, History and Examination*, 5e. London: W. B. Saunders.

Swartz, M. (2014). *Physical Diagnosis: History and Examination*, With Student Consult Online Access, 7e. London: Elsevier.

4 Examination of the Cardiovascular System

Carol Lynn Cox[1,2]
[1] *School of Health Sciences, City, University of London, London, UK*
[2] *Health and Hope Clinics, Pensacola, FL, USA*

4.1 Introduction

Examination of the cardiovascular system constitutes an essential aspect in evaluating the patient's health. Functions of the cardiovascular system involve the heart as a pump and the arteries and veins throughout the body in relation to transporting oxygen and nutrients to the tissues and transporting waste products and carbon dioxide from the tissues. Changes in the cardiovascular system affect other systems. The purpose of examining the cardiovascular system is to assess the function of the heart as a pump and arteries and veins throughout the body in transporting oxygen and nutrients to the tissues and transporting waste products and carbon dioxide from the tissues. Inspection, palpation, percussion, and auscultation are the key examination procedures implemented in this system.

Pocket Guide to Physical Assessment, First Edition. Edited by Carol Lynn Cox.

4.2 General Examination

In the narrative that follows, the essential elements associated with examination of the cardiovascular system are presented. Examination normally begins with history taking (subjective assessment), a review of systems (if not reviewed in association with a general physical examination), the objective examination, formation of a differential diagnosis, and diagnosis followed by a plan of treatment (Collins-Bride and Saxe 2013; Cox 2010; Crawford 2014; Jarvis 2008).

- Examine:
  - clubbing of fingernails
    Clubbing in relation to the heart suggests *cyanotic heart disease.*
  - cold hands with blue nails – poor perfusion, peripheral cyanosis
  - under the tongue, and at the gum line for central cyanosis (in light skinned patients the colour will be bluish purple, in dark skinned patients the colour will be grey)
  - conjunctivae for anaemia
  - signs of dyspnoea or distress
    Assess the degree of breathlessness by checking if *dyspnoea* occurs on undressing, talking, at rest, or when lying flat (*orthopnoea*).
  - xanthomata:
    - *xanthelasma* (common) – intracutaneous yellow cholesterol deposits occur around the eyes – normal or with *hyperlipidaemia*
    - *xanthoma* (uncommon)

hypercholesterolaemia – tendon deposits (hands and achilles tendon) or tuberous xanthomata at elbows

- *hypertriglyceridaemia* – eruptive xanthoma, small yellow deposits on buttocks and extensor surfaces, each with a red halo (Ball et al. 2014a, b; Barcauskas et al. 2002; Bickley and Szilagyi 2007, 2013; Cox 2010; Crawford 2014; Dains et al. 2012, 2015; Epstein et al. 2008; Hatton and Blackwood 2003; Japp and Robertson 2013; Jarvis 2015; Seidel et al. 2006, 2010; Swartz 2006, 2014; Talley and O'Connor 2006, 2014).

4.3 Palpate the Radial Pulse

Feel the radial pulse just medial to the radius with two forefingers.

Pulse rate:

Take for one minute (some clinicians will count the pulse for 15 seconds and multiply by four; however, this does not reflect an accurate pulse rate, particularly if the patient has arrhythmias):

- *tachycardia* > 100 beats min^{-1}
- *bradycardia* < 50 beats min^{-1}
- Rhythm:
  - regular

normal variation on breathing: *sinus arrhythmia*

- regularly irregular

pulsus bigeminus, coupled extrasystoles (digoxin toxicity)

Wenckebach (type I 2nd-degree heart block; the P–R interval lengthens until a P-wave is finally not conducted and the sequence starts again)

- irregularly irregular

atrial fibrillation

premature ventricular contractions (PVC), ventricular extrasystoles/ventricular ectopic beats (VE)

Check apical rate by auscultation whilst palpating the pulse for true heart rate, as ventricular premature beats are not transmitted to radial pulse (Crawford 2014; Fihn et al. 2012; Morse 2017).

- Waveform of the pulse:
  - normal (1)
  - slow rising and plateau – moderate or severe *aortic stenosis* (2)
  - collapsing pulse – pulse pressure greater than diastolic pressure, e.g. *aortic incompetence*, elderly *arteriosclerotic* patient or *gross anaemia* (3)
  - bisferiens – moderate *aortic stenosis* with severe *incompetence* (4)
  - pulsus paradoxus – pulse weaker or disappears on inspiration, e.g. *constrictive pericarditis, tamponade, status asthmaticus* (5) (Crawford 2014; Morse 2017).
- Volume:
  - small volume – *low cardiac output (CO)*
  - large volume

carbon dioxide retention
thyrotoxicosis (Crawford 2014; Morse 2017).

- Stiffness of the vessel wall:
  - In the elderly, a stiff, strongly pulsating, palpable 5–6 cm radial artery indicates *arteriosclerosis*, a hardening of the walls of the artery that:
  - is common with ageing
  - is not atheroma
  - is associated with systolic hypertension.
- Pulsus alternans:
  A difference of 20 mmHg systolic blood pressure (BP) between consecutive beats signifies poor left ventricular function. This needs to be measured with a sphygmomanometer (Crawford 2014; Morse 2017; Seidel et al. 2010; Swartz 2014; Talley and O'Connor 2014).

4.4 Take the Blood Pressure (BP)

Wrap the cuff neatly and tightly around either upper arm.

- Gently inflate the cuff until the radial artery is no longer palpable.
- Using the stethoscope, listen over the brachial artery for the pulse to appear as you drop the pressure slowly (3–4 mm s^{-1}).
- Systolic BP: appearance of sounds
  - Korotkoff phase 1
- Diastolic BP: disappearance of sounds
  - Korotkoff phase 5

Use large cuff for large arms (circumference > 30 cm) so that inflatable cuff >1/2 arm circumference.

Beware auscultatory gap with sounds disappearing mid-systole. If sounds go to zero, use Korotkoff phase 4.

In adults, ~> 140/85 mmHg or more is the current guideline in nondiabetic patients and ~> 130/80 mmHg in diabetic patients. The patient may be nervous when first examined and the BP may be falsely high. Take it again at the end of the examination.

Wide pulse pressure (e.g. 160/30 mmHg) suggests *aortic incompetence.*

Narrow pulse pressure (e.g. 95/80 mmHg) suggests *aortic stenosis.*

Difference of >20 mmHg systolic between arms suggests *arterial occlusion*, e.g. *dissecting aneurysm* or *atheroma*.

Difference of 10 mmHg is found in 25% of healthy subjects.

The variable pulse from atrial fibrillation means a precise BP cannot easily be obtained (Cox 2010; Dains et al. 2015; Fihn et al. 2012; Jarvis 2015; Morse 2017). Note that automated BP monitors will generally reflect higher readings than manual cuffs. If high readings are discerned with automated monitors it is recommended a manual BP be taken and recorded.

4.5 Jugular Venous Pulse (Frequently Called Pressure)

- Observe the height of the jugular venous pulsation (JVP).
  Position the patient lying at approximately 45° to the horizontal with head on pillows. Shine a torch at an angle across the neck.
- Look at the veins in the neck. Use tangential lighting.
  - internal jugular vein not directly visible: pulse diffuse, medial, or deep to sternomastoid
  - external jugular vein: pulse lateral to sternomastoid. Only informative if pulsating
- Assess vertical height in centimetres above the manubriosternal angle, using the pulsating external jugular vein or upper limit of internal jugular pulsation.

The external jugular vein is often more readily visible but may be obstructed by its tortuous course and is less reliable than the internal jugular pulse.

The internal jugular vein is sometimes very difficult to see. Its pulsation may be confused with the carotid artery but it:

- has a complex pulsation
- moves on respiration and decreases on inspiration except in tamponade
- cannot be palpated
- can be obliterated by pressure on base of neck
- demonstrates right heart pressure
  The hepatojugular reflux is checked by firm pressure with the flat of the right hand over the liver, whilst watching the JVP.
  Compression on the dilated hepatic veins increases the JVP by 2 cm.

If the JVP is found to be raised above the manubriosternal angle and pulsating, it implies *right heart failure*. Look for the other signs, i.e. pitting oedema and large tender liver. Sometimes the JVP is so raised it can be missed, except that the ears waggle.

Dilated neck veins with no pulsation suggest *noncardiac obstruction* (e.g. carcinoma bronchus causing superior caval obstruction or a kinked external jugular vein).

If venous pressure rises on inspiration (it normally falls), suspect *constrictive pericarditis* or *pericardial effusion* causing *tamponade* (Cox 2010; Crawford 2014).

- Observe the character of JVP. Try to ascertain the waveform of the JVP. It should be a double pulsation consisting of:
  - a-wave atrial contraction – ends synchronous with carotid artery pulse c
  - v-wave atrial filling – when the tricuspid valve is closed by ventricular contraction – with and just after carotid pulse

    Large a waves are caused by obstruction to flow from the right atrium due to stiffness of the RV from hypertrophy:
- *pulmonary hypertension*
- *pulmonary stenosis*
- *tricuspid stenosis.*

Absent a wave in *atrial fibrillation.*

Large v waves are caused by regurgitation of blood through an *incompetent tricuspid valve* during ventricular contraction.

A sharp y descent occurs in *constrictive pericarditis.*

Cannon waves (giant a waves) occur in *complete heart block* when the right atrium occasionally contracts against a closed tricuspid valve (Cox 2010; Crawford 2014).

4.6 Musset's Sign

- Observe the patient's ability to hold the head still.
  Slight rhythmic bobbing of the head in time with the heartbeat may accompany high back pressure caused by aortic insufficiency or aortic aneurysm (Cox 2010).

4.7 The Precordium

- Inspect the precordium for abnormal pulsation.
  A large LV may easily be seen on the left side of the chest, sometimes in the axilla.
- Palpate the apex beat (point of maximal impulse = PMI).
  - Feel for the point furthest out and down where the pulsation can still be distinctly felt. In the adult this is normally felt in the fifth intercostal space (ICS) midclavicular line (MCL). In the older adult this may shift to the sixth ICS just left of the MCL.
  - If you are unable to palpate the PMI, lean the patient forwards and turn the patient onto the left side. (This will slightly shift the heart forwards in the chest so that it is easier to feel.)
- Measure the position.
  - Determine the space, counting down from the second ICS which lies below the second rib (opposite the manubriosternal angle) where the PMI is felt.
  - Measure laterally in centimetres from the midline.
  - Describe the apex beat in relation to the MCL, anterior axillary line, and midaxillary line (Cox 2010).
- Assess character:

Try to judge if an enlarged heart is:

- feeble (dilated) or
- stronger than usual (LV or RV hypertrophy or both).

  Thrusting displaced apex beat occurs with volume overload: an active, large stroke volume ventricle, e.g. *mitral* or *aortic incompetence*, *left-to-right shunt* or *cardiomyopathy*.

  Sustained apex beat occurs with pressure overload in *aortic stenosis* and *gross hypertension*. Stroke volume is normal or reduced.

  Tapping apex beat (palpable first heart sound) occurs in *mitral stenosis*.

  Diffuse pulsation asynchronous with apex beat occurs with a *left ventricular aneurysm* – a dyskinetic apex beat.

  Impalpable – obesity, overinflated chest, pericardial effusion (Cox 2010; Bickley and Szilagyi 2013; Talley and O'Connor, 2014).

- Palpate firmly the left border of the sternum.
  - Use the flat of your hand.

    A heave suggests *right ventricular hypertrophy* (Cox 2010).
- Palpate all over the precordium with the flat of hand for thrills (palpable murmurs).

N.B. If by now you have found an abnormality in the cardiovascular system, think of possible causes before you listen.

For example, if LV is forceful:

- ? hypertension – was BP raised?
- ? aortic stenosis or incompetence – was pulse character normal? will there be a murmur?
- ? mitral incompetence – will there be a murmur?
- ? thyrotoxicosis or anaemia

4.8 Auscultation

- Listen over the five main areas of the heart and in each area with both the bell and diaphragm of the stethoscope.
  The bell will transmit soft sounds (S_3 and S_4) that are lost when the diaphragm is used. The diaphragm transmits loud harsh sounds. Concentrate in order on:
  - heart sounds
  - added sounds
  - murmurs.

Keep to this order when listening or describing what you have heard, or you will miss or forget important findings.

The five main areas are:

- apex, mitral area in the fifth ICS MCL (and left axilla if there is a murmur) = S_1 (Mitral = M_1)
- tricuspid area in the fourth ICS left sternal border = S_1 (Tricuspid = T_1)
- aortic area in the second ICS right of the sternum (and neck if there is a murmur) = S_2 (Aortic = A_2)
- pulmonary area in the second ICS left of the sternum = S_2 (Pulmonic = P_2)
- Erb's point in the third ICS left of the sternum = best location to hear murmurs across chambers

  These areas represent where heart sounds and murmurs associated with these valves are best heard. They do not represent the surface markings of the valves.

  If you hear little, turn the patient onto the left side, and listen over the apex (having palpated for it).

  Note that because the diaphragm filters out low-frequency sounds, the bell should be used for mitral stenosis, which is a low-frequency sound (Brown et al. 2002; Cox 2010).

4.8.1 Normal Heart Sounds

I Sudden cessation of mitral and tricuspid flow due to valve closure. (Use both the bell and diaphragm in auscultation.)

- loud in *mitral insufficiency (stenosis)*
- soft in *mitral incompetence, aortic insufficiency (stenosis), left bundle-branch block*
- variable in *complete heart block* and *atrial fibrillation*

II Sudden cessation of aortic and pulmonary flow due to valve closure – usually split (see below). (Use both the bell and diaphragm in auscultation.)

- loud in *hypertension*
- soft in *aortic* or *pulmonary insufficiency (stenosis)* (Heard best with the bell.)
- wide normal split – *right bundle-branch block*
- wide fixed split – *atrial septal defect* (Brown et al. 2002; Cox 2010).

4.8.2 Added Sounds

III First phase – rapid ventricular filling sound in early diastole (S_3). (Heard best with the bell lightly held. Pressure on the bell will extinguish the sound.)

- Common in children and young adults. In these instances it is known as a physiological S_3. It is heard in hyperkinetic states producing an increased CO. Examples include hyperthyroidism, exercise, pregnancy, and anxiety-related tachycardia. It can also be heard in mitral and tricuspid insufficiency, ischaemia, advanced congestive heart failure (CHF), and left to right shunts. When it is heard in middle-aged adults it is considered abnormal. You should suspect *left ventricular heart failure, fibrosed ventricle,* or *constrictive pericarditis*. When it originates in the LV it is best heard at the apex with patient on the left side exhaling. When it originates in the RV it is best heard at Erb's point (Brown et al. 2002; Cox 2010).

IV Second phase – atrial contraction (atrial kick) inducing ventricular filling towards the end of the diastole (S_4). (Heard best with the bell lightly held. Pressure on the bell will extinguish the sound.)

- A physiological S_4 may be heard in middle-aged adults who have thin-walled chests; especially after exercise. It occurs when there is an overload of either the LV or RV when diastolic pressure is increased. In the adult, suspect hyperthyroidism, pulmonary hypertension, aortic or pulmonary insufficiency, myocardial infarction (MI), or heart failure. In the older adult, suspect hypertensive cardiovascular disease, coronary artery disease, pulmonary hypertension, aortic or pulmonary insufficiency, myocardial ischaemia, infarction, or CHF. It may be the first evidence of cardiovascular disease. If it is heard over the left lateral sternal border it is probably RV in origin. If it is heard over the apex it is probably LV in origin (Brown et al. 2002; Cox 2010).

Canter rhythm (often termed gallop) with tachycardia gives the following cadences:

S_3: Frequently indicated as sounding like **Ken** – **tucky** (k = first heart sound). Note that S_3 comes after S_2.

S_4: Frequently indicated as sounding like **Tenne** – **ssee** (n = first heart sound) Note that S_4 comes before S_1 (Brown et al. 2002; Cox 2010).

4.8.3 Clicks and Snaps

- Normally the opening of a heart valve is silent. Ejection clicks arise from abnormal aortic or pulmonary valves when they open. These occur in early systole and may be mistaken as splitting. An opening snap (os) is associated with an abnormal mitral or tricuspid valve and is heard best in diastole (Brown et al. 2002; Cox 2010).

4.8.3.1 Opening Snap

- Mitral valve normally opens silently after S_2.
- In *mitral insufficiency (stenosis)*, sudden movement of rigid valve makes a snap, after S_2 (Brown et al. 2002; Cox 2010).

4.8.3.2 Ejection Click

- Aortic valve normally opens silently after S_1.
- In *aortic insufficiency (stenosis* or *sclerosis)*, the valve can open with a click after S_1 (Brown et al. 2002; Cox 2010).

4.8.4 Splitting of Second Heart Sound ($S_2 = a_2p_2$)

Ask patients to take deep breaths in and out. Blood is drawn into the thorax during inspiration and then on to the RV. There is temporarily more blood in the RV than the LV, and the RV takes fractionally longer to empty.

Splitting is best heard during inspiration. If the patient is breathless, do not ask them to hold breath in or out when assessing splitting.

Physiological splitting may occur in children and young people. In older people a delay in closure of $\mathbf{p}_2$ ($\mathbf{p}_2$ comes after $\mathbf{a}_2$) may be associated with right heart failure or pulmonary hypertension.

Paradoxical splitting occurs in *aortic insufficiency (stenosis)* and *left bundle-branch block.*

In both these conditions the LV takes longer to empty, thus delaying $\mathbf{a}_2$ until after $\mathbf{p}_2$. During inspiration $\mathbf{p}_2$ occurs later and the sounds draw closer together (Brown et al. 2002; Cox 2010).

4.8.5 Knock and Rub

A loud low-frequency diastolic noise best known as a knock can be heard in constrictive pericarditis. A pericardial friction rub is a high-pitched frequency noise, heard loudest in systole but frequently present in diastole as well. A rub may vary from hour to hour, and when a significant pericardial effusion occurs the rub will disappear (Brown et al. 2002; Cox 2010).

4.8.6 Murmurs

Use the diaphragm of the stethoscope for most high-pitched sounds or murmurs (e.g. aortic incompetence) and the bell for low-pitched murmurs (e.g. mitral insufficiency – stenosis). Note the following:

- Timing systolic or diastolic (compare with finger on carotid pulse).
- Site and radiation, e.g.:
  - mitral incompetence → axilla
  - aortic insufficiency (stenosis) → carotids and apex
  - aortic incompetence → sternum (Brown et al. 2002; Cox 2010).
- Character:
  - loud or soft
  - pitch, e.g. squeaking or rumbling, 'scratchy' = pericardial or pleural
  - length

    - pansystolic, throughout systole
    - early diastolic, e.g. aortic or pulmonary incompetence
    - midsystolic, e.g. aortic insufficiency (stenosis) or flow murmur
    - middiastolic, e.g. mitral insufficiency (stenosis) (Brown et al. 2002; Cox 2010)
- Relation to posture:
  - sit forwards – aortic incompetence louder
  - lie left side – mitral insufficiency (stenosis) louder
- Relation to respiration:
  - inspiration increases the murmur of a right heart lesion
  - expiration increases the murmur of a left heart lesion
  - variable – pericardial rub
- Relation to exercise:
  - increases the murmur of mitral insufficiency (stenosis) (Brown et al. 2002; Cox 2010)

4.8.6.1 Optimal Position for Hearing Murmurs

- Mitral insufficiency (stenosis) – the patient lies on left side, arm above head; listen with bell at apex as this is a diastolic murmur. Murmur is louder after exercise, e.g. repeated touching of toes from lying position that increases CO.
- Aortic incompetence (regurgitation) – the patient sits forwards after deep inspiration; listen with diaphragm at lower left sternal edge.

N.B. Murmurs alone do not make the diagnosis. Take other signs into consideration, e.g. arterial or venous pulses, BP, apex, or heart sounds. Also consider the status of the patient when deciding treatment. Does the patient look or state that they feel compromised? Is the patient breathless for example?

Loudness is often not proportional to severity of disease, and in some situations length of murmur is more important, e.g. mitral insufficiency (stenosis).

- For completion:
    - auscultate base of lungs for inspiratory and expiratory crackles from left ventricular failure
    - palpate liver – smooth, tender, enlarged in right heart failure
    - palpate peripheral pulses (? stronger in lower extremities than upper)
    - peripheral oedema – ankle/sacral (? right ventricular failure) (Cox 2010).

4.8.7 Summary of Timing of Murmurs

4.8.7.1 *Ejection Systolic Murmur*

- *aortic insufficiency (stenosis* or *sclerosis)* (same murmur, due to stiffness of valve cusps and aortic walls, with normal pulse pressure); *aortic insufficiency (sclerosis)* is present in 50% of 50-year-olds
- *pulmonary insufficiency (stenosis)*
- *atrial septal defect*
- *Fallot's syndrome* – right outflow tract obstruction

4.8.7.2 *Pansystolic Murmur*

- *mitral incompetence (regurgitation)*
- *tricuspid incompetence (regurgitation)*
- *ventricular septal defect*

4.8.7.3 *Late Systolic Murmur*

- *mitral valve prolapse – due to incompetence* (Frequently this sound is termed a systolic 'click')
- *hypertrophic cardiomyopathy*
- *coarction aorta* (extending in diastole to a 'machinery murmur')

4.8.7.4 Early Diastolic Murmur

- *aortic incompetence (regurgitation)*
- *pulmonary incompetence (regurgitation)*
- Graham Steell murmur in *pulmonary hypertension*

4.8.7.5 Mid–Late Diastolic Murmur

- *mitral insufficiency (stenosis)*
- *tricuspid insufficiency (stenosis)*
- Austin Flint murmur in *aortic incompetence*
- *left atrial myxoma* (variable – can also give other murmurs) (Cox 2010).

4.9 Signs of Left and Right Ventricular Failure

4.9.1 Left Heart Failure

- dyspnoea
- basal crackles on inspiration and expiration
- fourth heart sound (S4), or third in older patients (S3).
- Sit the patient forwards and listen at the bases of the lungs with the diaphragm of the stethoscope for fine inspiratory and expiratory crackles.

  Fine crackles heard on inspiration only are caused by alveoli opening on inspiration. If a patient has been recumbent for a while, alveoli tend to collapse in the normal lung. On taking a deep breath, fine inspiratory crackles will be heard. This is termed atelectasis. These do not mean the patient has fluid in the alveoli or pulmonary oedema. Ask the patient to take a deep breath and then cough. The crackles should clear. If crackles are present on inspiration and expiration, this is indicative of fluid in the alveoli. With medium to coarse crackles consider pulmonary oedema and request a chest X-ray for confirmation (Cox 2010).

4.9.2 Right Heart Failure

- raised JVP
- enlarged tender liver (see Chapter 6)
- pitting oedema
- With the patient sitting forwards, look for swelling over the sacral area. If there is, push your thumb into the swelling and see if you leave an indentation (pitting oedema). If you do, determine the severity of the oedema in terms of seconds it takes for the pitting to disappear.
- Check both ankles for pitting oedema.
  Oedema (fluid) collects at the most dependent part of the body. A patient who is mostly sitting will have ankle oedema whilst a patient who is lying will have predominantly sacral oedema (Cox 2010).

4.10 Functional Result

- Having ascertained the basic pathology (e.g. *MI, aortic insufficiency, stenosis, pericarditis*), make an assessment of the functional result.
  - history: how far can the patient walk, etc.
  - examination: evidence of:
    - cardiac enlargement (hypertrophy or dilatation)
    - heart failure
    - arrhythmias
    - pulmonary hypertension
    - cyanosis
    - endocarditis
  - investigations: for example:
    - chest X-ray
    - electrocardiogram (ECG/EKG)
    - treadmill exercise test with ECG/EKG for ischaemia

- echocardiograph – sonar 'radar' of heart, for muscle and ventricle size, muscle contractility and ejection fraction, valve function
- 24-hour ECG/EKG tape for arrhythmias
- cardiac catheterization for pressure measurements, blood oxygenation, and angiogram
- radioactive scan – to image live, ischaemic, or dead cardiac muscle (Cox 2010; Morse 2017).

4.11 Summary of Common Illnesses

4.11.1 Mitral Stenosis

- small pulse – fibrillating?
- JVP raised only if heart failure
- RV++ LVo tapping apex
- loud S_1; loud p_2 if pulmonary hypertension
- os
- middiastolic murmur at apex only (low-pitched rumbling)
    - severity indicated by early os and long murmur
    - best heard with the patient in left lateral position, in expiration with the bell of the stethoscope, particularly after exercise has increased CO
    - presystolic accentuation of murmur (absent if atrial fibrillation and stiff cusps)
- sounds 'ta ta rooofoo T'
- from S_2 os murmur S_1 (Cox 2010; Morse 2017).

4.11.2 Mitral Incompetence

- fibrillating?
- JVP raised only if heart failure
- RV+ LV++ systolic thrill
- soft S_1; loud p_2 if pulmonary hypertension
- pansystolic murmur apex → axilla (Cox 2010; Morse 2017).

4.11.3 Mitral Valve Prolapse

- midsystolic 'click', late systolic murmur
  - posterior cusp – murmur apex → axilla
  - anterior cusp – murmur apex → aortic area

4.11.4 Aortic Stenosis

- plateau pulse – narrow pulse pressure
- JVP raised only if heart failure
- LV++ systolic thrill
- soft a_2 with paradoxical split (± ejection click)
- harsh midsystolic murmur, apex and base, radiating to carotids
  - note discrepancy of forceful apex and feeble arterial pulse
- the longer the murmur, the tighter the stenosis; loudness does not necessarily imply severity (Cox 2010; Morse 2017).

4.11.5 Aortic Incompetence

- water-hammer pulse – wide pulse pressure; pulse visible in carotids
- JVP raised only if heart failure
- LV++ with dilatation

- (ejection click)
- early diastolic murmur base → lower sternum (also ejection systolic murmur from increased flow)
  - (sometimes Austin Flint murmur – see below)
  - heard best with patient leaning forwards, in expiration
- the longer the murmur, the more severe the regurgitation (Cox 2010; Morse 2017).

4.11.6 Tricuspid Incompetence

- JVP large v wave
- RV++, no thrill
- soft pansystolic murmur at maximal tricuspid area
- increases on inspiration (Cox 2010; Morse 2017).

4.11.7 Austin Flint Murmur

- middiastolic murmur (like mitral stenosis) in aortic incompetence due to regurgitant stream of blood on anterior cusp mitral valve

4.11.8 Graham Steell Murmur

- pulmonary early diastolic murmur (functional pulmonary incompetence) in mitral stenosis or other causes of pulmonary hypertension

4.11.9 Atrial Septal Defect

- JVP raised only if failure or tricuspid incompetence
- RV++ LVo
- widely fixed split-second sound
- pulmonary systolic murmur (tricuspid diastolic flow murmur) (Cox 2010; Morse 2017).

4.11.10 Ventricular Septal Defect

- RV+ LV+
- pansystolic murmur on left sternal edge (loud if small defect!)

4.11.11 Patent Ductus Arteriosus

- systolic → diastolic 'machinery' or continuous murmur below left clavicle

4.11.12 Metal Prosthetic Valves

- loud clicks with short flow murmur
  - aortic systolic
  - mitral diastolic
- need anticoagulation

4.11.13 Tissue Prosthetic Valves

- porcine xenograft or human homograft
- tend to fibrose after 7–10 years, leading to stenosis and incompetence
- may not require anticoagulation

4.11.14 Pericardial Rub

- scratchy (sounds like two pieces of leather rubbing together), superficial noise heard in systole and diastole
- brought out by stethoscope pressure, and sometimes variable with respiration (Cox 2010; Morse 2017).

4.11.15 Infectious Endocarditis (Diagnosis Made from Blood Cultures)

- febrile, unwell, anaemia
- splinter haemorrhages on nails
- Osler's nodes

- cardiac murmur
- splenomegaly
- haematuria

4.11.16 Rheumatic Fever

- flitting arthralgia
- erythema nodosum or erythema marginatum
- tachycardia
- murmurs
- *Sydenham's chorea* (irregular, uncontrollable jerks of limbs, tongue)

4.11.17 Clues to Diagnosis from Facial Appearance

- *Down's syndrome* from 21 trisomy
  - ventricular septal defect
  - patent ductus arteriosus
- *thyrotoxicosis* – atrial fibrillation
- *myxoedema* from hypothyroid – cardiomyopathy
- dusky, congested face – *superior vena cava obstruction*
- red cheeks in infra-orbital region in mitral facies from mitral stenosis

4.11.18 Clues to Diagnosis from General Appearance

- *Turner's syndrome* from sex chromosomes X0
  - female, short stature, web of neck
  - coarctation of aorta
- Marfan's syndrome
  - tall patient with long, thin fingers
  - aortic regurgitation (Hatton and Blackwood 2003; Cox 2010)

4.12 Peripheral Arteries

- Feel all peripheral pulses. Lower-limb pulses are usually felt after examining the abdomen.

  Diminished or absent pulses suggest *arterial stenosis* or *occlusion*. The lower-limb pulses are particularly important if there is a history of *intermittent claudication*.

  Auscultation of the carotid and femoral vessels is useful if there is a suspicion these arteries are stenosed. A bruit is heard if the stenosis causes turbulent flow.

  Coarctation of the aorta delays the femoral pulse after the radial pulse.

4.12.1 Peripheral Vascular Disease

- white or blue discoloration
- ulcers with little granulation tissue and slow healing
- shiny skin, loss of hairs, thickened dystrophic nails
- absent pulses
- Buerger's test of severity of arterial insufficiency
  - loss of autoregulation of blood flow
  - patient lying supine, lift leg up to 45° – positive test: pallor of foot; venous guttering (Cox 2010; Hatton and Blackwood 2003; Morse 2017).
  - hang legs over side of bed: note time to capillary and venous filling; reactive hyperaemia; subsequent cyanosis

    Diabetes, when present, also signs from neuropathy:
    - dry skin with thickened epidermis
    - callus from increased foot pressure over abnormal sites, e.g. under tarsal heads in midfoot, secondary to motor neuropathy, and change in distribution of weight
    - absent ankle reflexes
    - decreased sensation

4.12.2 Aortic Aneurysm

- Musset's sign (observe the patient's ability to hold the head still)
- central abdominal pulsation visible or palpable
- need to distinguish from normal, palpable aorta in midline in thin people
  - aortic aneurysm is expansible to each side as well as forwards
  - a systolic bruit may be audible
  - associated with femoral and popliteal artery aneurysms (Cox 2010; Hatton and Blackwood 2003; Morse 2017).

4.13 Varicose Veins

- Varicose veins and hernia are examined when the patient is standing, possibly at the end of the whole examination at the same time as the gait. Majority are associated with incompetent valves in the long saphenous vein or short saphenous vein.

  Long saphenous – from femoral vein in groin to medial side of lower leg.

  Short saphenous – from popliteal fossa to back of calf and lateral malleolus.
- Observe:
  - swelling
  - pigmentation – indicates chronic venous insufficiency
  - eczema
  - inflammation – suggests thrombophlebitis
- Palpate:
  - soft or hard (thrombosed)
  - tender – thrombophlebitis
  - cough impulse – implies incompetent valves

Incompetent valves can be confirmed by the Trendelenburg test:

- Elevate leg to empty veins.
- Occlude long saphenous vein with a tourniquet around upper thigh.
- Stand patient up.
- If veins fill rapidly, this indicates incompetent thigh perforators below the tourniquet.
- If, after release of tourniquet, veins fill rapidly, this indicates incompetent saphenofemoral junction.

If veins fill immediately on standing, then incompetent valves are in thigh or calf, so do the Perthes test:

- As for Trendelenburg, but on standing let some blood enter veins by temporary release of groin pressure.
- Ask patient to stand up and down on toes.
- Veins become less tense if:
    - muscle pump is satisfactory
- perforating calf veins are patent with competent valves (Cox 2010; Hatton and Blackwood 2003; Morse 2017).

4.14 System Orientated Examination

4.14.1 'Examine the Cardiovascular System'

- hands –? moist, cold clammy, palmar erythema
- nails – leukonychia, splinter haemorrhages, capillary refill

- radial pulse – rate, rhythm, waveform, volume, state of artery
- BP
- eyes – anaemia
- area around eyes – xanthelasma
- mouth – central cyanosis
- JVP – height, waveform
- apex beat – PMI site, character
- auscultate
    - at apex – PMI (with thumb/finger on carotid artery for timing)
        - heart sounds
        - added sounds
        - murmurs
    - in neck over carotid artery – each area of precordium with diaphragm
        - aortic incompetence – lean forwards in full expiration with diaphragm
        - mitral stenosis – lay patient on left side and listen at apex with bell
- listen to the bases of lungs for crackles
- examine for hepatomegaly
- peripheral oedema and peripheral pulses (Ball et al. 2014a,b; Barcauskas et al. 2002; Bickley and Szilagyi 2007, 2013; Cox 2010; Crawford 2014; Dains et al. 2012, 2015; Epstein et al. 2008; Hatton and Blackwood 2003; Japp and Robertson 2013; Jarvis 2015; Seidel et al. 2006, 2010; Swartz 2006, 2014; Talley and O'Connor 2006, 2014).

4.15 Reference Guide: Intracardiac Values and Pressures

See Table 4.1.

Table 4.1 Intracardiac values and pressures.

Intracardiac values	
Cardiac output (CO)	4–8 l min^{-1}
Cardiac index (CI)	2.4–4.2 l min^{-1} m^{-2}
Stroke volume (SV)	60–120 ml
Stroke volume index (SVI)	35–70 ml $beat^{-1}$ m^{-2}
Left cardiac work (LCW)/left cardiac work index (LCWI)	3.4–4.2 kg m m^{-2}
Left ventricular stroke work (LVSW)/ left ventricular stroke work index (LVSWI)	LVSW = 50–60 g-m m^{-2}
right cardiac work (RCW)/right cardiac work index (RCWI)	RCW = 0.54–0.66 km-m m^{-2}
Right ventricular stroke work (RVSW)/ right ventricular stroke work index (RVSWI)	RVSWI = 7.9–9.7 g-m m^{-2}
Systemic vascular resistance (SVR)	900–1600 dyn s^{-1} cm^{-5}
Pulmonary vascular resistance (VR)	20–120 dyn s^{-1} cm^{-5}
Mixed venous saturation (SvO_2)	75%
Delivery of oxygen (DO_2)	900–1100 ml min^{-1}
Consumption of oxygen (VO_2)	200–290 ml min^{-1}
Oxygen extraction ratio (OER)	0.22–0.30
Intracardiac pressures	
Central venous pressure (CVP)	0 – +8 mmHg (right atrial level)
Right ventricle (RV)	0 – +8 mmHg diastolic
	+15 – +30 mmHg systolic
Pulmonary capillary wedge pressure (PCWP)	
	+5 – +15 mmHg
Left atrium (LA)	+4 – +12 mmHg
Left ventricle (LV)	+4 – +12 mmHg diastolic
	+90 – +140 mmHg systolic
Aorta	+90 – +140 mmHg systolic
	+60 – +90 mmHg diastolic
	+70 – +105 mmHg mean

References

Ball, J., Dains, J., Flynn, J. et al. (2014a). *Seidel's Guide to Physical Examination*, 8e. St. Louis: Mosby.

Ball, J., Dains, J., Flynn, J. et al. (2014b). *Student Laboratory Manual to Accompany Seidel's Guide to Physical Examination*, 8e. St. Louis: Mosby.

Barkauskas, V., Baumann, L., and Darling-Fisher, C. (2002). *Health and Physical Assessment*, 3e. London: Mosby.

Bickley, L. and Szilagyi, P. (2007). *Bates' Guide to Physical Examination and History Taking*, 9e. Philadelphia: Lippincott.

Bickley, L. and Szilagyi, P. (2013). *Bates' Guide to Physical Examination and History Taking*, 11e. New York: Wolters Kluwer/Lippincott Williams & Wilkins.

Brown, E., Collis, W., Leung, T., and Salmon, A. (2002). *Heart Sounds Made Easy*. Edinburgh: Churchill Livingstone.

Collins-Bride, G. and Saxe, J. (2013). *Clinical Guidelines for Advanced Practice Nursing – An Interdisciplinary Approach*, 2e. Burlington, MA: Jones and Bartlett Learning.

Cox, C. (2010). *Physical Assessment for Nurses*, 2e. Oxford: Wiley Blackwell.

Crawford, M. (2014). *Current Diagnosis and Treatment: Cardiology*, 4e. New York: McGraw-Hill Education.

Dains, J., Baumann, L., and Scheibel, P. (2012). *Advanced Health Assessment and Clinical Diagnosis in Primary Care*, 4e. St. Louis: Elsevier.

Dains, J., Baumann, L., and Scheibel, P. (2015). *Advanced Health Assessment and Clinical Diagnosis in Primary Care*, 5e. St. Louis: Mosby.

Epstein, O., Perkin, G., de Bono, D., and Cookson, J. (2008). *Clinical Examination*, 4e. London: Mosby.

Fihn, S., Gardin, M., Abrama, J. et al. (2012). Guideline for the diagnosis and management of patients with stable ischemic heart disease. *J. Am. Coll. Cardiol.* 60 (24): 1–121.

Hatton, C. and Blackwood, R. (2003). *Lecture Notes on Clinical Skills*, 4e. Oxford: Blackwell Science.

Japp, A. and Robertson, C. (2013). *Macleod's Clinical Diagnosis*. Edinburgh: Churchill Livingstone, Elsevier.

Jarvis, C. (2008). *Physical Examination and Health Assessment*, 5e. St. Louis: Saunders.

Jarvis, C. (2015). *Physical Examination and Health Assessment*, 7e. Edinburgh: Elsevier.

Morse, C. (2017). Cardiovascular System. In: *Family Nurse Practitioner & Adult-Gerontology Nurse Practitioner* (ed. A. Rundio and W. Lorman), 99–118. New York: Wolters Kluwer.

Seidel, H., Ball, J., Dains, J., and Benedict, G. (2006). *Mosby's Physical Examination Handbook*. St. Louis: Mosby.

Seidel, H., Ball, J., Dains, J., and Benedict, G. (2010). *Mosby's Physical Examination Handbook*, 7e. St. Louis: Mosby-Year Book.

Swartz, M. (2006). *Physical Diagnosis, History and Examination*, 5e. London: W. B. Saunders.

Swartz, M. (2014). *Physical Diagnosis: History and Examination*, With Student Consult Online Access, 7e. London: Elsevier.

Talley, N. and O'Connor, S. (2006). *Clinical Examination: A Systematic Guide to Physical Diagnosis*, 5e. London: Churchill Livingstone.

Talley, N. and O'Connor, S. (2014). *Clinical Examination: A Systematic Guide to Physical Diagnosis*, 7e. London: Churchill Livingstone, Elsevier.

5

Examination of the Respiratory System

Carol Lynn Cox[1,2]
[1]School of Health Sciences, City, University of London, London, UK
[2]Health and Hope Clinics, Pensacola, FL, USA

5.1 Introduction

The respiratory assessment constitutes an essential aspect in evaluating the patient's health. Functions of the respiratory system involve the exchange of oxygen and carbon dioxide in the lungs and tissues and regulation of the acid–base balance. Changes in the respiratory system affect other systems. Inspection, palpation, percussion, and auscultation are the key examination procedures implemented in this system.

5.2 General Examination

- Examine the patient for:
  - signs of respiratory distress (tachypnoea, dyspnoea, nasal flaring, use of accessory muscles, cyanosis, patient leans forwards and uses pursed lip breathing, inability to speak without pausing)
  - nicotine on fingers, fingernails, and along the hairline in light haired individuals

Pocket Guide to Physical Assessment, First Edition. Edited by Carol Lynn Cox.

- clubbing: respiratory causes include:
    - intrathoracic tumours:
      carcinoma of bronchus
      mesothelioma
      cystic fibrosis
    - bronchiectasis
    - lung abscess
    - empyema
    - fibrosing alveolitis
    - chronic obstructive pulmonary disease (COPD) (e.g. emphysema)
    - mixed venous to arterial shunts
    - chronic hepatic fibrosis
- evidence of respiratory failure:
    - hypoxia: central cyanosis, seen on the lips, tongue (versus peripheral cyanosis seen on the fingers and nail beds)
    - hypercapnia: drowsiness, confusion, papilloedema, warm hands, bounding pulse, dilated veins, coarse tremor/flap
- respiratory rate: count per minute (note normal or abnormal rate)
- pattern of respiration:
- Cheyne–Stokes (causes):
    - alternating hyperventilation and apnoea
    - severe increased intracranial pressure of the brainstem
    - left ventricular failure
    - high altitude
    - congestive heart failure
    - uremia
- Biot's – ataxic breathing:
    - unpredictable irregularity (respirations may be shallow or deep and are interrupted by periods of apnoea – seen in neurologic disease/disorders)

- hyperventilation or Kussmaul respiration:
  - increases in both rate and depth (hyperpnoea is an increase in depth only – seen in exercise, anxiety, and metabolic acidosis; Kussmaul is hyperventilation associated with metabolic acidosis)
- tachypnoea:
  - rapid, shallow breathing >24 breaths per minute (seen in restrictive lung disease, pleuritic chest pain, elevated diaphragm, acute illnesses, and pneumonia)
- air trapping:
  - present in pulmonary diseases (as air is trapped in the lungs, respiratory rate rises and breathing becomes shallow)
- positional dyspnoea
  - orthopnoea: inability to lie flat when breathing. The individual must sit or stand in order to breathe deeply or comfortably. (seen in congestive heart failure, severe asthma, emphysema, mitral valve disease, chronic bronchitis, neurologic disease)
  - trepopnoea: dyspnoea when lying on one side but not on the other – lateral recumbent position. (seen in congestive heart failure: patient is more comfortable breathing whilst lying on one side)
  - platypnoea: shortness of breath (breathlessness) that is relieved when lying down and worsens when sitting or standing up. It is the opposite of orthopnoea. (seen in neurologic disease, cirrhosis causing intrapulmonary shunts, hypovolaemia, status post pneumonectomy)

- obstructive airways disease:
    - pursed-lip breathing:
        - expiration against partially closed lips
    - chronic obstructive airways disease to delayed closure of bronchioles
    - use of accessory muscles:
        - sternomastoids
        - strap muscles and platysma muscles
- wheezing (Consider inspiratory versus expiratory.):
    - bronchospasm
    - asthma (crackles and rhonchi)
    - allergy
    - congestive heart failure
    - tumour
    - obstruction (wheezing/respiratory sounds are absent below the obstruction)
    - chronic obstructive pulmonic disease
- stridor: partial obstruction of trachea
    - hoarse voice:
        - abnormal vocal cords
        - or recurrent laryngeal palsy
- cough:
    - haemoptysis (coughing up blood)
    - sputum production (chronic/productive related to chronic bronchitis, bronchiectasis, abscess, bacterial pneumonia, tuberculosis)
    - dry/hacking (viral infection, interstitial lung disease, allergies, tumour)
    - barking (epiglottal disease such as croup)
    - morning ('smoker's cough')
    - nocturnal (postnasal drip, congestive heart failure)

    - when eating or drinking (neuromuscular disease of the upper oesophagus)
  - sleep apnoea: characterised by daytime fatigue, sleepiness, disruptive snoring, episodic upper airway obstruction, nocturnal hypoxemia (Ball et al. 2014a, b; Barkauskas et al. 2002; Bickley and Szilagyi 2013; Cox 2010; Hatton and Blackwood 2003; Kacmarck et al. 2017; Swartz 2006, 2014).

First examine the front of the chest fully and then similarly examine the back of the chest.

- Landmarks to locate the lungs):
  - manubrium of the sternum
  - sternal angle (angle of Louis)
  - sternum
  - xiphoid process
  - sternal notch or jugular notch
  - costal angle
  - clavicles
  - scapulae
  - spinous processes
  - acromial processes (Ball et al. 2014a, b; Barkauskas et al. 2002; Bickley and Szilagyi 2013; Cox 2010; Hatton and Blackwood 2003; Japp and Robertson 2013; Jarvis 2008, 2015; Swartz 2006, 2014)
- Demarcation lines of the thorax:
  - used to identify and describe the location/condition of underlying organs/sounds

5.3 Physical Assessment of the Chest

- Examination of the chest

Examination of the chest involves inspection, palpation, percussion, and auscultation. When inspecting, palpating, percussing, and auscultating, the chest terminology for charting a normal examination should reflect:

On inspection – 'breathing without difficulty' or 'normal BBS' (bilateral breath sounds).
On palpation – 'no TTP' (tenderness to palpation).
On percussion – 'clear to percussion bilaterally'.
On auscultation – 'CTAB' (clear to auscultation bilaterally) (Cox 2010).

5.4 Inspection of the Chest

- Rest the patient comfortably in the bed or examination couch/table at 45°:
  - compare hemithoraces; progress from the neck down
  - distended neck, puffy blue face and arms
  - superior mediastinal obstruction
  - tracheal shift (Cox 2010; Rhoads and Paterson 2013; Seidel et al. 2006, 2010; Talley and O'Connor 2006, 2014; Tallia and Scherger 2013)
- Inspect the shape of the chest:
  - colour, contour, and condition of the skin (ecchymosis, lesions, scars, e.g. from previous surgery)
  - asymmetry: diminution of one side or possible flail
  - lung collapse
  - fibrosis
  - deformity: check spine (Scoliosis: C or S curve often at the level of the thoracic spine; Kyphosis: curvature of the cervical spine forwards – flexion)

- pectus excavatum: sunken sternum (congenital abnormality)
- pectus carinatum: 'pigeon breast' (congenital abnormality)
- barrel chest (increased anterior and posterior diameter)
- obstructive airways disease
- barrel chest: lower costal recession on deep inspiration; cricoid cartilage close to sternal notch; chest appears to be fixed in inspiration (Bickley and Szilagyi 2013; Cox 2010; Hatton and Blackwood 2003; Swartz 2006, 2014; Talley and O'Connor 2006, 2014).

5.5 Palpation

- Check integrity of the thorax (palpate ribs, clavicles, sternum, and scapulae for abnormalities):
  - crepitations (e.g. fracture or unstable sternum; also palpable under the skin in pneumothorax)
  - pain (over ribs in fracture versus over intercostal spaces in costochrondritis)
- Check mediastinum position:
  - trachea – check position: palpate with a single finger in the midline and determine if it slips preferentially to one side or the other
- Lymph nodes, supraclavicular fossae/axillae – *tuberculosis, lymphoma, cancer of the bronchus*, cancer of the breast, infraclavicular and parasternal
- Apex beat – may be displaced because of enlarged heart and not a shift in the mediastinum

  Unequal movement of chest:
  - Look from the end of the examination table/couch or bed
  - Classic method of palpation to discern respiratory excursion:

  - extend your fingers – anchor fingertips far laterally around chest wall whilst your extended thumbs meet in the midline
  - on inspiration, assess whether there is asymmetrical movement of thumbs from midline (movement should be equal 1–2 cm)
- Alternative method of palpation to discern respiratory excursion:
  - lay a hand comfortably on either side of the chest and, using these as a gauge, assess if there is diminution of movement on one side during inspiration

N.B. Diminution of movement on one side indicates pathology on that side. In older adults, respiratory excursion may be minimal to absent as anterior–posterior dimension of the thorax develops and lateral movement diminishes (Bickley and Szilagyi 2013; Cox 2010).

- Palpate intercostal spaces for abnormalities:
  - lumps, surgical emphysema
- Tactile fremitus:
  - vocal fremitus (assessed when pathology is suspected) (Cox 2010).

5.6 Percussion

- Percuss with the middle finger (hammer finger) of one hand against the middle phalanx of the middle finger of the other, laid flat on the chest. The hammer finger should strike at right angles and the wrist of the hammer finger hand should flick with each strike. See Table 5.1 for discrimination of sounds.

Table 5.1 Discrimination of sounds.

Sound	Relative intensity	Relative pitch	Relative duration
Flatness	Soft	High	Short
Dullness	Medium	Medium	Medium
Resonance	Loud	Low	Long
Hyperresonance	Very loud	Lower	Longer
Tympani	Loud	Hollow	Hollow

- Percuss both sides of the chest for resonance, at top, middle, and lower segments. Compare sides, and if different also compare the front and back of chest.
- If a dull area exists, map out its limits by percussing from a resonant to the dull area.
- Percuss the level of the diaphragm from above downwards.

  Increased resonance may occur in:
  - pneumothorax
  - emphysema.

  Decreased resonance may occur in:
  - *effusion:* very dull – sometimes called stony dullness
  - *solid lung*
    - consolidation
    - alveolar collapse
    - abscess
  - neoplasm.

Remember the surface markings of the lungs when percussing. Thus, the lower lobe predominates posteriorly and the upper lobe predominates anteriorly (Bickley and Szilagyi 2013; Cox 2010; Hatton and Blackwood 2003; Swartz 2006, 2014; Talley and O'Connor 2006, 2014).

- Determine diaphragmatic excursion by percussing the level of the diaphragm from above downwards. Start with the patient breathing normally. Percuss downwards from the bottom of the scapula in the intercostal spaces from tympani to dullness. When dullness is heard, mark this space. Ask the patient to take a deep breath and hold it. Percuss from the marked space (tympani) to dullness. Diaphragmatic excursion should be greater on the left than on the right. (Position of the liver diminishes excursion on the right. Position of the heart increases excursion on the left.)
  - *decrease in excursion indicative of diaphragmatic paralysis (seen following cardiothoracic surgery and abdominal surgery or trauma/injury)*

5.7 Auscultation

- Before listening, ask patient to cough up any sputum, which may create adventitious sounds.
- Use either the diaphragm or bell of the stethoscope, dependent on the condition/physique of the patient, and listen starting at the top (apex), middle, and bottom (base) of both sides of the chest, and then in the axilla. Auscultate downwards in approximately 5 cm distances.

Ask the patient to breathe through the mouth moderately deeply. It helps to demonstrate this yourself (Cox 2010).

The bell of the stethoscope is used to hear low-pitched sounds. Hold the bell lightly on the patient's skin. If pressure is put on the bell, a diaphragm will be created and the ability to hear low-pitched sounds will be lost. In cachectic, thin patients, patients with prominent ribs or if the chest is hairy, use of the bell is more effective. Protruding ribs make placement of the stethoscope diaphragm difficult as pressure must be applied to the diaphragm in order to use it effectively (Swartz 2006, 2014).

It is not acceptable to listen to the chest through clothing as some soft sounds may be lost. The bell/diaphragm must always be in direct contact with the patient's skin.

- Listen for normal breath sounds (Table 5.2), comparing both sides:
  - vesicular: breath sounds heard over most of the lung tissue
  - bronchovesicular: heard near the bronchi (e.g. below the clavicles and between the scapulae, especially on the right)
  - bronchial: patent bronchi plus conducting tissue
  - tracheal/tubular: sounds similar to sounds with stethoscope over trachea
- Listen for added sounds (adventitious sounds), and note if inspiratory or expiratory
  - tracheal/tubular or bronchial: sounds heard in an area other than the upper or lower trachea
    - consolidation (usually pneumonia)
    - *neoplasm*
    - *fibrosis*
    - *abscess*
  - diminution: indicates either no air movement (e.g. obstructed bronchus) or air or fluid preventing sound conduction
    - effusion
    - pneumothorax
    - emphysema (early sign is atelectasis)
    - collapse – obstruction (absent breath sounds)
  - crackle (outdated terms include rales, crepitations and creps): caused by either the alveoli popping open on inspiration (indicative of atelectasis) or fluid in the lungs (in which the

Table 5.2 Characteristics of sounds.

Breath sound	Duration of inspiration and expiration	Pitch of expiration	Intensity of expiration	Sample location
Vesicular	Inspiration longer than expiration	Low	Soft	Most of lungs
Bronchovesicular	Inspiration and expiration are equal	Medium	Medium	Near bronchi, e.g. below the clavicles and between the scapulae, especially on the right
Bronchial	Expiration longer than inspiration	Medium-high (dependent on location)	Usually high (dependent on location)	Over the lower part of the trachea
Tracheal/tubular	Expiration longer than inspiration	High	High/harsh	Over the upper part of the trachea

crackling sound is heard on inspiration and expiration)
    - fine – heart failure, alveolitis, or if late on inspiration indicative of pulmonary fibrosis
    - medium – infection or fluid in the alveoli
    - coarse – air bubbling through fluid in the alveoli and larger bronchioles, e.g. bronchiectasis or pulmonary oedema
- pulmonary fibrosis (delayed crackles on inspiration – late on inspiration)
- wheeze (outdated terms include sibilant rale, musical rale, sonorous rale or low-pitched wheeze): caused by rapid airflow through a constricted airway (Consider whether the wheeze is inspiratory, expiratory, or both.)
    - asthma – note the presence of air trapping
    - COPD – note the presence of air trapping
    - bronchitis
    - cystic fibrosis
    - pulmonary oedema
    - congestive heart failure
- rhonchus: transient airway plugging caused by mucous secretions
    - bronchitis
- pleural rub: caused by *pleurisy* (inflammation of the pleura due to pneumonia or pulmonary infarction); sounds like two pieces of leather rubbing together
- stridor: high pitched sound on inspiratory caused by turbulent airflow through narrowed trachea (considered a medical emergency in epiglottitis, croup, and allergic reactions) (Bickley and Szilagyi 2013; Collins-Bride and Saxe 2013; Cox 2010; Epstein et al. 2008; Hatton and Blackwood 2003; Swartz 2006, 2014; Talley and O'Connor 2006, 2014).

5.8 Vocal Fremitus/Resonance

Should be assessed by using the ulnar surface of your hands to feel for increased vibrations when pathology is suspected.

Speech creates vibrations that can be evaluated through feeling and hearing. The presence or absence of fremitus can provide useful information about the density of underlying lung tissue and the chest cavity. Conditions that increase density increase the transmission/frequency of tactile fremitus. Conditions that decrease the transmission of sound waves decrease tactile fremitus.

- Ask the patient to repeat '99' whilst you palpate the patient's chest with either the ulnar surface or palms of both of your hands simultaneously in the same general areas as auscultation. The frequency of vibrations is greater over areas of consolidation. Compare both sides.
- You can also auscultate for vocal resonance. Ask the patient to say 'e'.
- At the surface of an *effusion* the word 'e' takes on a bleating character like a goat, which is called aegophony. If vocal resonance is gross, whispered pectoriloquy can be elicited by asking the patient to whisper: '1, 2, 3' repeatedly. The whispered sound when auscultated will be loud and pronounced rather than soft and muffled (Bickley and Szilagyi 2013; Cox 2010; Hatton and Blackwood 2003; Swartz 2006, 2014; Talley and O'Connor 2006, 2014).

N.B. Vocal fremitus, breath sounds, and vocal resonance all depend on the same criteria and vary together.

To determine further clues check:

- chest movement asymmetry
- mediastinum displacement
- percussion

(Barkauskas et al. 2002; Bickley and Szilagyi 2007; Epstein et al. 2008; Hatton and Blackwood 2003; Jarvis 2008, 2015; Seidel et al. 2006; Swartz 2006, 2014; Talley and O'Connor 2006, 2015; Tallia and Scherger 2013).

5.9 Sputum

Examination of the sputum is unpleasant but important. Normally 75–100 ml of sputum is secreted daily by the bronchi.

Describe according to colour, consistency, quantity, presence or absence of blood or pus, and number of times brought up during the day and night.

- Look for:
  - colour (yellow or green suspect mucus; rust colour is from R/T enzyme release from neutrophils which occur in viruses and/or bacteria – suspect infection but this cannot be confirmed without a culture) (Tallia and Scherger 2013)
  - consistency
  - quantity (increased grossly in bronchiectasis)
  - blood (cancer, tuberculosis, embolus).
- Ideally the sputum should be examined under the microscope for:
  - bacteria
  - pus cells
  - eosinophils
  - plugs
  - asbestos (Cox 2010; Epstein et al. 2008).

5.10 Functional Result

- Make an assessment of the functional result:
  - history – exertion/exercise: for example, how far can the patient walk and how many stairs can be climbed

- examination:
  - $P\text{o}_2$ ↓: central cyanosis
    - confusion
  - $P\text{co}_2$ ↑: peripheral signs
    - warm periphery
    - dilated veins
    - bounding pulse
    - flapping tremor
  - central signs
    - drowsy
    - papilloedema
    - small pupils
- Check by arterial blood gases.
- Tests (usually undertaken for COPD):
  - force of expiration: blowing out a lighted match about 15 cm from the mouth and with the mouth wide open is easy as long as the patient's peak flow is above approximately $80\,\text{l}\,\text{min}^{-1}$ (normal $300\text{–}500\,\text{l}\,\text{min}^{-1}$)
  - expiration time: an assessment of airways obstruction can be made by timing the period of full expiration through wide-open mouth following a deep breath; this should be less than two seconds when normal
  - chest expansion: expansion from full inspiration to full expiration should be more than 5 cm; reduced if hyperinflation of the chest is due to chronic obstructive airways disease
  - peak flow: a measure of airways obstruction is the peak rate of flow of air out of the lungs; a record is made using a peak flow meter; normal $300\text{–}500\,\text{l}\,\text{min}^{-1}$
  - spirometry: standard test for diagnosis (Cox 2010).

5.11 Summary of Common Illnesses

5.11.1 Asthma

- patient distressed, tachypnoeic, unable to talk easily
- wheeze on expiration audible or by auscultation
- overinflated chest with hyperresonance
- if central cyanosis: critically ill, artificial ventilation?
- pulsus paradoxus (variation in systolic pressure during inspiration and expiration and may be normal between attacks)
- often due to atopy
- enquire about exposure to antigens:
    - house dust mite
    - cats or dogs
    - chemical exposure (Cox 2010).

5.11.2 Pneumonia

- inflammatory condition affecting the alveoli

5.11.3 Bronchitis

- inflammation of the bronchi

5.11.4 Bronchiectasis

- chronic condition in which the walls of the bronchi are thickened from inflammation and infection of the bronchi

5.11.5 Obstructive Airways Disease (Chronic)

- also termed COPD (chronic obstructive pulmonary disease)
- barrel chest

- accessory muscles of respiration in use
- hyperresonance
- depressed diaphragm – indrawing lower costal margin on inspiration
- diminished breath sounds:
    - blue bloater:
        - central cyanosis
        - signs of carbon dioxide retention
        - obese
        - not dyspnoeic
        - ankle oedema: may or may not have right heart failure
    - pink puffer:
        - not cyanosed
        - no carbon dioxide retention
        - thin
        - dyspnoeic
        - no oedema

5.11.6 Bronchiectasis

- abnormal widening and thickening of the bronchi and/or branches
- clubbing
- constant green/yellow phlegm
- coarse crackles over affected area

5.11.7 Allergic Alveolitis

- extrinsic – seen in farmer's lung; mushroom picker's disease; humidifier or air-conditioner lung; bird breeder's or bird fancier's lung. Diagnosed through images and bronchoscopy
- clubbing
- fine, unexplained crackles, widespread over bases (Cox 2010).

5.12 System-Oriented Examination

5.12.1 'Examination of the Respiratory System'

Use the techniques of inspection, palpation, percussion, and auscultation in each phase of the examination whilst examining the anterior, posterior, and lateral thorax.

- hands: clubbing, signs of increased carbon dioxide (warm hands, bounding pulse, coarse tremor)
- face: nasal flaring
- tongue: central cyanosis
- trachea: right or left shift
- supraclavicular, infraclavicular, and parasternal nodes
- inspection
  - shape of chest contour
  - chest movements
  - respiration rate/rhythm/depth/distress
  - colour and condition of the skin
- palpation
  - interspaces for abnormalities
  - sternum, ribs, clavicles, and scapulae for abnormalities
  - excursion
  - vocal fremitus
- percussion: in 5 cm intervals from apex to base – upper segments (L, R), middle (L, R) and lower segments (L, R)
  - diaphragmatic excursion
- auscultation:
  - breath sounds
  - added sounds (adventitious sounds)
- if COPD:
  - expiration time (Cox 2010; Dains et al. 2012, 2015).

References

Ball, J., Dains, J., Flynn, J. et al. (2014a). *Seidel's Guide to Physical Examination*, 8e. St. Louis: Mosby.

Ball, J., Dains, J., Flynn, J. et al. (2014b). *Student Laboratory Manual to Accompany Seidel's Guide to Physical Examination*, 8e. St. Louis: Mosby.

Barkauskas, V., Baumann, L., and Darling-Fisher, C. (2002). *Health and Physical Assessment*, 3e. London: Mosby.

Bickley, L. and Szilagyi, P. (2007). *Bates' Guide to Physical Examination and History Taking*, 9e. Philadelphia: Lippincott.

Bickley, L. and Szilagyi, P. (2013). *Bates' Guide to Physical Examination and History Taking*, 11e. New York: Wolters Kluwer/Lippincott Williams & Wilkins.

Collins-Bride, G. and Saxe, J. (2013). *Clinical Guidelines for Advanced Practice Nursing – An Interdisciplinary Approach*, 2e. Burlington, MA: Jones and Bartlett Learning.

Cox, C. (2010). *Physical Assessment for Nurses*, 2e. Oxford: Wiley Blackwell.

Dains, J., Baumann, L., and Scheibel, P. (2012). *Advanced Health Assessment and Clinical Diagnosis in Primary Care*, 4e. St Louis: Elsevier.

Dains, J., Baumann, L., and Scheibel, P. (2015). *Advanced Health Assessment and Clinical Diagnosis in Primary Care*, 5e. St. Louis: Mosby.

Epstein, O., Perkin, G., de Bono, D., and Cookson, J. (2008). *Clinical Examination*, 4e. London: Mosby.

Hatton, C. and Blackwood, R. (2003). *Lecture Notes on Clinical Skills*, 4e. Oxford: Blackwell Science.

Japp, A. and Robertson, C. (2013). *Macleod's Clinical Diagnosis*. Edinburgh: Churchill Livingstone, Elsevier.

Jarvis, C. (2008). *Physical Examination and Health Assessment*, 5e. St. Louis: Saunders.

Jarvis, C. (2015). *Physical Examination and Health Assessment*, 7e. Edinburgh: Elsevier.

Kacmarek, R., Stoller, J., and Heuer, A. (2017). *Egan's Fundamentals of Respiratory Care*, 11e. St. Louis: Mosby.

Rhoads, J. and Paterson, S. (2013). *Advanced Health Assessment and Diagnostic Reasoning*, 2e. Burlington: Jones and Bartlett.

Seidel, H., Ball, J., Dains, J., and Benedict, G. (2006). *Mosby's Physical Examination Handbook*. St. Louis: Mosby.

Seidel, H., Ball, J., Dains, J., and Benedict, G. (2010). *Mosby's Physical Examination Handbook*, 7e. St. Louis: Mosby-Year Book.

Swartz, M. (2006). *Physical Diagnosis, History and Examination*, 5e. London: W. B. Saunders.

Swartz, M. (2014). *Physical Diagnosis: History and Examination*, With Student Consult Online Access, 7e. London: Elsevier.

Talley, N. and O'Connor, S. (2006). *Clinical Examination: A Systematic Guide to Physical Diagnosis*, 5e. London: Churchill Livingstone.

Talley, N. and O'Connor, S. (2014). *Clinical Examination: A Systematic Guide to Physical Diagnosis*, 7e. London: Churchill Livingstone, Elsevier.

Talley, N. and O'Connor, S. (2015). *Clinical Examination*, 8e. Edinburgh: Churchill Livingstone.

Tallia, A. and Scherger, J. (2013). *Swanson's Family Practice Review*, 6e. St Louis: Mosby.

6

Examination of the Abdomen

Anthony McGrath
London South Bank University, London, UK

6.1 Introduction

An abdominal assessment constitutes an essential aspect in evaluating the patient's health. Changes in the function of organs within the abdomen affect other systems. By understanding the role and function of the GI tract you are better placed to understand the signs and symptoms exhibited in abdominal disease as well as having a firmer grasp of the organs you are examining during the examination. Inspection, auscultation, palpation, and percussion are the key examination procedures implemented in this system.

6.2 General Examination

Before commencing your abdominal examination, introduce yourself to the patient as this will allow you to establish a rapport and allow you to identify the patient to be examined.

- ensure privacy and the patient's dignity by screening the examination couch/table/bed by closing the curtains and/or the door.

Pocket Guide to Physical Assessment, First Edition. Edited by Carol Lynn Cox.

- ensure the patient can be assessed in good light as this will allow you a better opportunity to note any abnormalities (Amico and Barbarito 2016; McGrath 2010).
- to conduct a detailed assessment the patient will need to be exposed from the nipples to the knees.
- maintain the patient's dignity by covering them with a sheet as much as possible.
- inform the patient of what you are going to do
- obtain their consent prior to commencing the examination.
- stand on the patient's right as this will enable you to easily determine the span of the liver (Amico and Barbarito 2016; Ball et al. 2014a, b; Bickley and Szilagyi 2013; McGrath 2010; Ranson et al. 2014; Thomas and Monaghan 2014).

Your history should have alerted you to any specific problems that you will need to explore further such as dyspepsia, vomiting, dysphagia, pain, bleeding, or an altered bowel habit. The symptoms and signs noted in GI disease usually reflect disorders in the main abdominal organs (McGrath 2010).

6.3 Abdominal Pain

Pain is probably one of the most significant symptoms in abdominal problems and whilst it will vary greatly depending on the cause, by carefully considering the nature of pain you can gain some insight as to what may be wrong with the patient.

- Visceral pain is caused by increased tension on the splanchnic nerves contained in the muscular wall. It is common in obstructive lesions and it is sometimes colicky in type.

- Referred pain is usually caused by the abdominal viscera being irritated by an inflamed organ or a neoplasm.
- Peritoneal pain is associated with a deep tenderness and often with muscular rigidity.
- As part of your assessment you need to consider the character of the pain.
- mild discomfort or is it severe
- what aggravates or relives the pain.
- Duration
- whether it comes on after or before meals (*pain that is of short duration is more likely due to an obstructive cause*)
- associated symptoms such as nausea and vomiting, sweating, or a temperature (Ball et al. 2014a, b; Bickley and Szilagyi 2013; Dains et al. 2012, 2015; Douglas et al. 2013; Japp and Robertson 2013; Ranson et al. 2014; Talley and O'Connor 2013; Thomas and Monaghan 2014).

Before you begin your examination, it is important for the patient to be relaxed as much as possible as tense muscles will hinder your examination. Ensure that the room is warm. Ask the patient to empty their bladder. This has a twofold effect: (i) it will make them more comfortable and (ii) it allows you the opportunity to test the urine. Ask the patient to lie flat, arms loosely by their sides and their head resting on a pillow, as this will allow the abdominal muscles to relax. By propping another pillow under the patient's knees, the patient is more comfortable (McGrath 2010). Do not allow the patient to place their hands above their heads as this action stretches and tightens the abdominal wall making examination more difficult (Ball et al. 2014a, b; Bickley and Szilagyi 2013; Douglas et al. 2013; Epstein et al. 2008; Japp and Robertson 2013; Jarvis 2015; McGrath 2010; Ranson et al. 2014; Thomas and Monaghan 2014).

The examination should follow a straightforward format.

- Inspection (Examine the entire abdomen by looking from the foot of the bed initially for the shape of the abdomen. Is it convex or concave? The normal abdomen is concave and symmetrical. The normal abdomen is concave and symmetrical. It will rise and fall in line with respiration. Look for signs of peristalsis. Then progress to examine the abdomen by looking from the right and left side of the patient.)
- Auscultation (Note that in examination of the abdomen it is important to auscultate before percussing and palpating as percussion and palpation can alter bowel sounds.)
- Percussion (Listen for tympanic sounds and dull sounds which indicate the presence of air (tympany) and solid organs or tumours (dull/flat sounds)
- Palpation (Feel for the presence of organs in their normal position. Are there irregularities in position or is softness, hardness or sharp edges present?)

6.4 Inspection

Conduct a systematic inspection of the patient. This involves a generalised inspection followed by a more detailed inspection. Any abnormalities detected on inspection will provide clues to any underlying pathology which can be investigated further during auscultation, percussion, and palpation. Before beginning the inspection take and record the patient's pulse and note its rate and regularity. A tachycardia may suggest infection or internal bleeding whereas atrial fibrillation may be linked to emboli lodging in the mesenteric arteries which in turn can lead to bowel ischaemia and the patient presenting with severe abdominal pain (Ball et al. 2014a, b; Bickley and Szilagyi 2013; Douglas et al. 2013; Epstein et al. 2008; Japp and Robertson 2013; Jarvis 2015; Ranson et al. 2014; Talley and O'Connor 2013; Thomas and Monaghan 2014).

To begin the inspection:

- Consider whether the patient look well or unwell
- note the skin colour and condition. (Is the skin jaundiced, dry, or bruised or does it have scratch marks?)

Inspection involves:

- noting the presence of any surgical scars as these may provide information regarding previous pathology.
- noting whether the patient has striae (stretch marks). Note the colour. If silvery in appearance this can be due to the patient previously losing weight or a result of pregnancy. Striae that are purplish/pink and wider may be indicative of Cushing's syndrome which is caused by the excessive secretion of cortisol (Bickley and Szilagyi 2013; Douglas et al. 2013; Jarvis 2015; McGrath 2010; Ranson et al. 2014; Talley and O'Connor 2013; Thomas and Monaghan 2014).
- squatting down so that you can view the abdomen tangentially. (You will need to do this from both sides. It is important that you do this in good light. In this position you can more easily pick out subtle changes of shadow and contour. Asymmetrical movement may indicate the presence of a mass.)
- inspecting the patient's face and then work your way down the body. (If the patient is jaundiced this is best seen in the sclera and in the oral mucosa.)
- inspecting the eyes note the presence of Kayser-Fleischer rings. (These are brownish-greenish rings which are visible at the periphery of the cornea. They are caused by copper deposits and a sign of Wilson's disease.)
- looking at the conjunctivae for signs of anaemia. (*A distinctly pale conjunctiva is frequently a sign that the patient has a haemoglobin of 9 or less.*)

- looking for the presence of brown freckles 1–5 mm in diameter on lips or buccal mucosa which may indicate Peutz–Jeghers syndrome. The freckles can also be seen on fingers; another feature of this syndrome is polyps in the small bowel that can give rise to abdominal pain, bleed, or intussusception or become malignant (Ball et al. 2014a, b; Bickley and Szilagyi 2013; Dains et al. 2015; Douglas et al. 2013; Jarvis 2015; Ranson et al. 2014; Talley and O'Connor 2013; Thomas and Monaghan 2014).
- looking for the presence of telangiectasia, which are small, widened blood vessels on the skin. They are usually harmless and have been associated with sun exposure. However, they are also linked with poor flow to the vessels and may be caused by alcohol abuse, pregnancy, and ageing. They can also be found in the intestines, which can bleed.
- looking (with a pen torch/pen light/small flashlight) around and inside the mouth. A dry tongue may be indicative of 'dehydration' or mouth-breathing. If the patient appears dehydrated, check for Maxwell's sign (lift fold of skin on forehead above the nose between the eyebrows). The skin fold remains raised in patients who are dehydrated. Look at the lips – are they cracked or sore? Reddish brown cracks radiating from the corners of the mouth are indicative of angular stomatitis, which is caused by vitamin B6, B12, folate, and iron deficiency (Bickley and Szilagyi 2013; Japp and Robertson 2013; Jarvis 2015; McGrath 2010; Ranson et al. 2014; Talley and O'Connor 2013; Thomas and Monaghan 2014).
- noting the colour of the lips and mouth. (If cyanosis is seen it is important to determine if it is peripheral or central. Simply ask the patient to stick out their tongue. If the tongue is a normal colour and moist, then the patient has peripheral cyanosis. You need to

warm them up. However, if the tongue and mucosa are discoloured (blue to purple in colour) it may be indicative of central cyanosis or chronic liver disease from pulmonary arteriovenous shunting [Ball et al. 2014a, b; Bickley and Szilagyi 2013; Douglas et al. 2013; Jarvis 2015; Ranson et al. 2014; Talley and O'Connor 2013; Thomas and Monaghan 2014]).

- noting the presence of a red tongue and whether it has creamy white curdlike patches (This is indicative of candidiasis. However, if you do note white coloured lesions on the tongue or in the mouth this may be due to leukoplakia, which is a premalignant condition. The presence of glossitis which presents as a smooth red tongue is indicative of B12, folate, and iron deficiency. Note that in patients with B12 or folate deficiency the tongue is painful whereas in iron deficiency the patient experiences no pain [McGrath 2010]).
- noting any breath odours (These can be indicative of underlying problems. A faecal smell may be linked to obstruction, whereas patients with hepatic failure may have a sickly sweet odour on their breath. The presence of an alcohol smell may indicate the need to explore for liver problems [Ball et al. 2014a, b; Bickley and Szilagyi 2013; Thomas and Monaghan 2014]).
- noting any gingivitis or ulcers inside the mouth. (In patients with Crohn's disease ulcers may be seen at the corners of the mouth or they may be caused by ill-fitting dentures. Poor dental hygiene may also lead to gingivitis. Furring of the tongue can occur in patients who smoke, are taking antibiotics, or have GI problems [Thomas and Monaghan 2014]).
- Looking at the neck and noting the presence of any enlarged nodes in the left supraclavicular fossa which may indicate a malignancy in the GI tract.

(A hard node felt behind the left sternoclavicular joint may be a Virchow's node and suggests an abdominal neoplasm spread by lymphatics via the thoracic duct. A large left supraclavicular node in association with carcinoma of the stomach is known as Troisier's sign [Bickley and Szilagyi 2013; Douglas et al. 2013; Jarvis 2015; Thomas and Monaghan 2014]).

- Looking at the chest. (Is there the normal distribution of hair? Males with liver disease may present with gynaecomastia. Also in males, poor hair distribution over the trunk is linked with patients with alcoholic liver disease. Patients with liver disease may also present with a loss of axillary and chest hair. Bear in mind the current fashion of removing body hair.)
- noting the presence of spider naevi (Dilated blood vessels that are linked to pregnancy, malnutrition, and liver disease. In pregnancy they usually appear between the second and third trimesters and usually disappear following the birth. However, the presence of more than five of them is considered abnormal and may be linked to cirrhosis [Bickley and Szilagyi 2013; Douglas et al. 2013; Jarvis 2015; Thomas and Monaghan 2014]).

(As noted previously, normally, the abdomen is concave and symmetrical and moves gently with respiration. However, if the abdomen is distended this may be due to one of the five Fs: flatus, faeces, foetus, fat, or fluid. Localised swellings may indicate the enlargement of an abdominal or pelvic organ. If a swelling is noted, try to determine if it moves with or is independent of respiration. Bulging around scars may indicate the presence of an incisional hernia [Bickley and Szilagyi 2013; Douglas et al. 2013; Jarvis 2015; Thomas and Monaghan 2014]).

- noting the presence of any dilated or engorged veins in the abdominal wall. (Veins are rarely prominent in healthy individuals. If they can be seen it is important to determine whether it is abnormal or not. This can be done by determining the flow of blood within the vein. Place two fingers onto the vein. By doing this the flow of blood is prevented. Slide one finger along the vein thus creating a gap between your two fingers. By doing this the vein is emptied. Now lift the finger you slid away from the other finger and observe. If the vein refills determine the direction the blood flows. If the blood flow below the umbilicus flows up towards the umbilicus it may be due to inferior vena cava obstruction. If the flow of blood is downwards away from the umbilicus this may be due to portal vein hypertension [Bickley and Szilagyi 2013; Douglas et al. 2013; Epstein et al. 2008; Jarvis 2015; McGrath 2010; Thomas and Monaghan 2014]).
- noting peristalsis. (If there is visible peristalsis this is not usually normal. However, it may be visible in very thin patients. Demonstrative [hyperactive] peristalsis can be indicative of pyloric obstruction or obstruction of the distal small intestine. If you think it is a possible pyloric obstruction you will need to test for a succession splash. To do this, first make sure that the patient has been nil by mouth for at least three hours. Once this has been established gently shake the patient's abdomen by holding either side of the pelvis. If you hear a splashing noise either with the naked ear or with the chest piece of a stereoscope placed just above the umbilicus, this is a positive sign. The patient is likely to have a pyloric obstruction [Bickley and Szilagyi 2013; Douglas et al. 2013; Jarvis 2015; McGrath 2010; Thomas and Monaghan 2014]).

- noting the presence of an expansile pulsation in the epigastric region. (This may be caused by an aortic aneurysm. If the patient is aged 60 years or more, smokes, and has hypertension consider this if you note a pulsation in the abdomen [McGrath 2010]).
- noting discoloration on the abdominal wall. (A bluish discoloration or ecchymosis in either the flank [Grey Turner's sign] or around the periumbilical area [Cullen's sign] is caused by the seepage of blood-stained ascetic fluid into the subcutaneous tissue and is seen in acute haemorrhagic pancreatitis or a retroperitoneal haemorrhage.)
- looking for the presence of a hernia in the umbilical region. (The umbilicus is normally located within 1 cm of the midpoint between the xiphoid and the symphysis pubis. Any deviation of more than 1 cm required palpation in this area as it may be displaced by an underlying mass [Bickley and Szilagyi 2013; Jarvis 2015; Thomas and Monaghan 2014]).
- examining the hands

  for signs of palmar erythema (Although it can be a normal finding it is usually found in pregnancy and in chronic liver disease.)

  for signs of Dupuytren's contracture (A visible and palpable thickening and contraction of the palmar fascia. It causes a permanent flexion and is generally associated with alcohol abuse; however, it can also be found in manual workers.)

  for signs of clubbing in the fingers (Caused by inflammatory bowel disease or coeliac disease.)

  for signs of liver flap (asterixis) when the patient holds their arms outstretched with their wrists dorsiflexed for a minimum of 20 seconds. (A liver flap is an irregular coarse tremor that occurs in liver failure (Bickley and Szilagyi 2013; Jarvis 2015; Thomas and Monaghan 2014).

for any signs of pitting, ribbing, and brittleness in the nails, which are linked to malabsorption syndromes. (The presence of koilonychia [spoon-shaped spongy nails] are indicative of iron deficiency anaemia. Leukonychia or white nails occurs in liver failure or hypoalbuminaemia.)
- checking the arms for bruising or scratch marks (Excessive bruising may indicate a clotting abnormality and scratch marks suggest that the patient has pruritus, which is symptom of cholestatic jaundice [McGrath 2010]).

6.5 Auscultation

Auscultation will provide information about bowel motility. Therefore, it is important to listen to the bowel before performing palpation or percussion as they can alter the frequency of bowel sounds. Bowel sounds are caused by intestinal peristalsis moving gas and fluid through the bowel. Place the diaphragm of the stereoscope on the abdomen. Listen over the abdomen for about 10–15 seconds. If sounds are difficult to hear listen for up to seven minutes. Normal bowel sound can be heard as gurgles and clicks. Borborygmi are prolonged gurgling sounds, the sounds you hear when your stomach rumbles (Bickley and Szilagyi 2013; Jarvis 2015; Thomas and Monaghan 2014).

In progressive bowel obstruction large amounts of fluid and gas accumulate and hyperactive 'tinkling' bowel sounds can be heard. This is an ominous sign of impending bowel paralysis. Paralytic ileus or generalised peritonitis gives complete absence of bowel sounds. Listen for hepatic bruits in patients with liver disease. A soft and distant bruit heard over an enlarged liver is always abnormal and may indicate primary liver cell cancer, alcoholic hepatitis, or acquired arteriovenous shunts from biopsy or trauma (Bickley and Szilagyi 2013; Jarvis 2015; Thomas and Monaghan 2014).

6.5.1 Arterial Bruits

If appropriate from the history or examination (e.g. the patient has high blood pressure), listen for bruits over the renal, iliac, and femoral arteries. Renal arteries are sometimes best heard over the back. Renal artery stenosis may be the cause of hypertension. Patients with intermittent claudication may have flow bruits over the femoral arteries from narrowing, e.g. atheroma (McGrath 2010).

6.6 Palpation

Ensure your hands are warm. Tell the patient to inform you if it hurts when you begin to palpate. In order to elicit the most information, it is important that palpation is conducted in two stages: first, light palpation. This will allow identification of any tenderness and second, deep palpation which will allow for the detection of deeper masses. It also allows for any masses previously found to be defined.

Before feeling or palpating the patient's abdomen ask:

- 'Is your abdomen painful anywhere?' Get the patient to point to where the pain is worst.
- 'Does the pain radiates anywhere?' Consider its onset and duration.

To begin lightly palpate 1–3 cm in depth in each quadrant, starting away from the site of pain or tenderness. Your hand should be flat on the patient's abdomen. Palpate in nine quadrants (Refer to Chapter 2). Palpate each abdominal quadrant in turn using the palmar surface of the fingers as this will allow you to mould your hand to the shape of the abdominal wall. Be gentle. As you palpate look at the patient's face to see if palpation is hurting the patient or causing any discomfort. Note any tenderness which may be superficial, deep, or rebound. Rebound tenderness will be exhibited when inflamed viscera in peritonitis move against the parietal peritoneum. Note any guarding, which is a voluntary muscle spasm to protect from pain. The patient may lie on their side with knees flexed to prevent stretching of the abdominal wall. In peritonitis, for example, stretching of the abdominal wall causes the patient to experience pain (McGrath 2010).

Now perform deeper palpation. Press deeply 4–6 cm and evenly into the abdominal wall. Muscle rigidity along with distention is suggestive of peritonitis. As you palpate the abdomen note any masses and if a mass is found, describe the site, size, shape, consistency (e.g. faeces may be indented by pressure), fixation, or mobility. Does it move on respiration? Note if it is tender or pulsatile, which is the transmitted pulsation from the aorta or pulsatile swelling. Note if it is dull to percussion. This is particularly important to determine if bowel is in front of mass. Note if the mass is present after defecation or micturition.

6.6.1 Liver and Gall Bladder

Now palpate for the liver edge. Start about 10 cm below the costal margin and work up towards the ribs. You can use your fingertips or two hands or if you prefer the radial side of your index finger on one hand. Ask the patient to take a deep breath. As the patient takes a deep breath press your fingers inwards and upwards. At the height of the patient's inspiration slightly relax your inward pressure whilst maintaining the upward pressure. The liver should descend and as it does so, the liver edge should slide under your fingers. In healthy individuals the liver edge can usually be palpated just below the costal margin. Describe position of liver edge in centimetres below the costal margin of the midclavicular line. Liver enlargement is described as mild, moderate, or massive. If enlarged, feel the shape of liver edge to determine whether the edge is firm or hard, regular/irregular, tender, or pulsatile (in tricuspid incompetence). If the liver is large remember to palpate for the spleen as the presence of a palpable spleen suggests cirrhosis with portal hypertension. Percuss the upper and lower borders of liver after palpation to confirm findings (Bickley and Szilagyi 2013; Jarvis 2015; McGrath 2010; Thomas and Monaghan 2014).

Conclude your liver palpation by feeling for the gall bladder. The fundus can normally be found where the rectus muscle intersects with the costal margin (tip of ninth costal cartilage). Ask the patient to take a deep breath and using the tips of your fingers, apply firm pressure. If the gall bladder is inflamed the patient will exhibit tenderness, guarding, and intense pain as your fingers make contact with the gall bladder (Murphy's sign). If your patient has jaundice and the gall bladder is palpable then the cause is most likely to be a malignancy (Courvoisier's law).

6.6.2 Spleen

The normal spleen cannot be felt and becomes palpable only when it has doubled/trebled in size. Ask the patient to take deep breaths, as air-filled lungs push the spleen down, so it can be palpated. Roll the patient onto their right side with his left arm hanging loosely in front as your examining hand is gently worked up towards the left costal margin. If the spleen is not palpable, percuss area for splenic dullness. The spleen can be enlarged to the hypogastrium. Common causes of splenomegaly include portal hypotension, malaria, haemolytic anaemia, and leukaemia. If you can feel the spleen it is important to note the size and shape (Can you feel the splenic notch?); whether you can feel above it or whether it moves on respiration. You will describe your findings as you do for the liver (Bickley and Szilagyi 2013; Jarvis 2015; McGrath 2010; Thomas and Monaghan 2014).

6.6.3 Groin

Now palpate the spermatic cord, lymph nodes, and arteries that occupy the groin. Swellings here are usually caused by hernias or enlarged lymph nodes. Palpate the groin to detect enlarged lymph nodes. Most people have small, shotty nodes. Most enlarged tender nodes arise from infection in the legs or feet. However, in some Afro-Caribbean men this is normal. If large nodes are felt, palpate the spleen carefully (reticulosis or leukaemia) (McGrath 2010).

6.6.4 Hernia

When checking for the presence of a hernia examine the patient standing and ask them to cough. An enlargement of a swelling in the groin is highly suggestive of a hernia. With an indirect (oblique) inguinal hernia the swelling can be reduced to the internal inguinal ring by applying pressure on the contents of hernial sac and then controlled by pressure over the internal ring when the patient is asked to cough. When your hand is removed, the impulse passes medially towards the external ring and is palpable above the pubic tubercle. In patients with a direct inguinal hernia the impulse is felt in a forward direction mainly above the groin crease medial to the femoral artery. Swelling is not controlled by pressure over the internal ring (Bickley and Szilagyi 2013; Jarvis 2015; McGrath 2010; Thomas and Monaghan 2014).

6.6.5 Kidneys and Bladder

The kidneys are difficult to feel. Deep bimanual palpation is required to explore them. This is achieved by placing one hand under the back and the other on the front of the loin. Ask the patient to take deep breaths as you ballot the kidney. As they do so push up with left hand in the renal angle and feel kidney anteriorly with right hand (this is termed 'cupping'). Getting the patient to take a deep breath will bring the kidneys between your hands. A common sign of infection is tenderness over the kidneys. The presence of a large kidney may indicate a tumour (e.g. polycystic disease or hydronephrosis). To assess further for kidney tenderness, you can check for costal-vertebral angle tenderness. Ask the patient to sit forwards and place the palm of your hand over the renal angle. Then using the ulnar surface of your other hand, make a fist and strike your hand placed on the patient's renal angle with moderate force. Perform on each kidney in turn and assess the patient's reaction. This should not cause any pain unless there is some inflammation of the kidney (McGrath 2010).

Palpate for the bladder in the hypogastric area and if a mass is found, percuss to confirm the presence of fluid. If the patient is suffering from urinary retention a full bladder may be felt above the pubic symphysis. As you palpate the patient will feel uncomfortable and will want to pass urine. Therefore, ensure your patient has emptied their bladder before you perform this manoeuvre.

6.6.6 Aorta

Palpate in the midline above the umbilicus for a pulsatile mass. If easily palpated, suspect aortic aneurysm and proceed to ultrasonography in males over 60 and women over 65 years. As you inspect the patient note any bobbing of the head with each pulsation of the aorta (de Musset's sign). De Musset's sign is indicative of coarctation of the aorta. Refer to Chapter 4, Examination of the Cardiovascular System, for more information regarding this sign.

6.7 Percussion

It is important to percuss all four quadrants for dullness and tympany (Refer to Chapter 2). Good percussion technique will allow you to assess the amount and distribution of gas in the abdomen. It will also allow you to determine the size of the liver and spleen. Dull sounds are normal over solid organs; however, any dull sound is abnormal is the middle of the abdomen. If dullness is noted in areas other than over a solid organ note the presence of ascites and consider a possible cause such as a mass (e.g. large ovarian cyst). Percuss over liver, spleen, and kidneys and percuss over any suspected mass. The midline of the abdomen should be resonant. If not, think of gastric neoplasm, omental secondaries, enlarged bladder, ovarian cyst, pregnancy. If you note a generalised swelling or distention of the abdomen lay the patient on one side and mark the upper level of dullness. Roll the patient flat and see if the level shifts. If it does, this is referred to as shifting dullness. Note that in ascites there is central tympani and lateral dullness. In ovarian tumour, there is central dullness and lateral tympani as the gas-filled bowel is pushed laterally (McGrath 2010).

6.8 Examination of Genitals

Ask in a sensitive way before you proceed. For example, 'I should briefly examine you down below. Is that all right?' In the male, palpate the scrotum for the testes and epididymis. It is rarely necessary to examine the penis unless the patient complains of a rash, discharge, or ulceration. However, tender and enlarged testes may occur with orchitis or torsion of the testis. A large, soft swelling which transilluminates suggests hydrocele or an epididymal cyst. A hydrocele surrounds the testis; an epididymal cyst lies behind the testis. A large, hard, painless testis suggests cancer. On inspection of the penis if you note the presence of balanitis (inflamed glans of penis) this should remind you to check for diabetes (McGrath 2010).

6.9 Digital Rectum Examination

- Tell the patient at each stage what you are going to do.
- Lay the patient on the left side with knees flexed to the chest.
- Say: 'I am going to put a finger into your back passage'.
- Inspect the anus for lumps, haemorrhoids, fissures, ulcers, inflammation, excoriation, and discolouration. A bluish discolouration of perineal skin may be indicative of Crohn's disease.
- With lubricant on the examination glove, press your fingertip against the anal verge then gently slip your forefinger into the anal canal and then into the rectum. Feel the tone of the sphincter by asking the patient to squeeze your finger with their anal muscles; then check the size and character of the prostate and any lateral masses. If appropriate, proceed to proctoscopy.
- Test stool on your glove for occult blood.

6.10 Per Vaginam Examination

- Tell the patient at each stage what you are going to do.
- Lay the patient on her left side as for per rectum examination (although some nurses prefer the patient lying on her back with hips flexed and knees abducted. Note that this position is difficult for the older adult to maintain and uncomfortable.)
- Inspect the external genitalia.
- With lubricant on the examination glove insert one finger into vagina and then a second finger if there is room. (If a smear must be taken, this should be done before bimanual palpation is undertaken.)
- Palpate the cervix (check for cervical excitation, which is present in pelvic inflammatory disease).
- Examine for the position and enlargement of the uterus, tenderness of appendages and masses.
- Check for discharge by observing the glove.

6.11 Summary of Common Illnesses

6.11.1 Cirrhosis

- leukonychia
- clubbing
- palmar erythema
- spider naevi
- jaundice
- firm liver

6.11.2 Portal Hypertension

- splenomegaly
- ascites
- caput medusa

6.11.3 Hepatic Encephalopathy

- liver flap
- drowsy
- constructional apraxia (cannot draw five-pointed star)
- musty fetor

6.11.4 'Dehydration' (Water and Salt Loss)

- dry skin
- veins collapsed
- diminished skin turgor – pinched fold of skin on forehead remains raised (Maxwell's sign)
- tongue dry
- eyes sunken
- blood pressure low with postural drop

6.11.5 Intestinal Obstruction

- patient 'dehydrated' if they have been vomiting
- abdomen centrally swelling
- visible peristalsis
- not tender (unless inflammation or some other pathology)
- resonant to percussion
- high-pitched 'tinkling' bowel sounds

6.11.6 Pyloric Stenosis

- otherwise like intestinal obstruction
- may have 'succussion splash' on shaking abdomen
- upper abdomen swelling

6.11.7 Appendicitis

- slight fever
- deep tenderness right iliac fossa or per rectum-
- otherwise little to find unless has spread to peritonitis

6.11.8 Peritonitis

- lies still
- abdomen:
    - does not move on respiration
    - rigid on palpation (guarding)
    - tender, particularly on removing fingers rapidly (rebound tenderness)
- absent bowel sounds
- tender right hypochondrium, particularly on breathing in (Murphy's sign – tender gall bladder descends on inspiration to touch your palpating hand)

6.11.9 Jaundice and Palpable Gall Bladder

- obstruction is not due to gallstones but from another obstruction such as neoplasm of the pancreas (Courvoisier's law); gallstones have usually caused a fibrosed gall bladder which cannot dilate from back pressure from gallstones in common bile duct

6.11.10 Enlarged Spleen

- infective, e.g. septicaemia or subacute bacterial endocarditis
- portal hypertension, e.g. cirrhosis
- lymphoma
- leukaemia and other haematological diseases
- autoimmune, e.g. systemic lupus, Felty's syndrome

References

Amico, D. and Barbarito, C. (eds.) (2016). *Health and Physical Assessment in Nursing*. New Jersey: Prentice Hall.

Ball, J., Dains, J., Flynn, J. et al. (2014a). *Seidel's Guide to Physical Examination*, 8e. St. Louis: Mosby.

Ball, J., Dains, J., Flynn, J. et al. (2014b). *Student Laboratory Manual to Accompany Seidel's Guide to Physical Examination*, 8e. St. Louis: Mosby.

Bickley, L. and Szilagyi, P. (2013). *Bates' Guide to Physical Examination and History Taking*, 11e. New York: Lippincott, Williams and Wilkins.

Dains, J., Baumann, L., and Scheibel, P. (2012). *Advanced Health Assessment and Clinical Diagnosis in Primary Care*, 4e. St Louis: Elsevier.

Dains, J., Baumann, L., and Scheibel, P. (2015). *Advanced Health Assessment and Clinical Diagnosis in Primary Care*, 5e. St. Louis: Mosby.

Douglas, G., Nichol, F., and Robertson, C. (eds.) (2013). *Macleod's Clinical Examination*. Edinburgh: Churchill Livingston.

Epstein, O., Perkin, G., de Bono, D., and Cookson, J. (2008). *Clinical Examination*, 4e. London: Mosby.

Japp, A. and Robertson, C. (2013). *Macleod's Clinical Diagnosis*. Edinburgh: Churchill Livingstone, Elsevier.

Jarvis, C. (2015). *Physical Examination and Health Assessment*, 7e. Edinburgh: Elsevier.

McGrath, A. (2010). Examination of the abdomen. In: *Physical Assessment for Nurses*, 2e (ed. C. McGrath), 101–112. Oxford: Wiley Blackwell.

Ranson, M., Braithwaite, W., and Abbott, H. (eds.) (2014). *Clinical Examination Skills for Healthcare Professionals*. Cumbria: MK Publishing.

Talley, N. and O'Connor, S. (2013). *Clinical Examination: A Systematic Guide to Physical Diagnosis*, 7e. Oxford: Blackwell Science.

Thomas, J. and Monaghan, T. (eds.) (2014). *Oxford Handbook of Clinical Examination and Practical Skills*, 2e. Oxford: Oxford University Press.

7

Examination of the Male Genitalia

Carol Lynn Cox[1,2] *and Anthony McGrath*[3]

[1] *School of Health Sciences, City, University of London, London, UK*
[2] *Health and Hope Clinics, Pensacola, FL, USA*
[3] *London South Bank University, London, UK*

7.1 Introduction

Research indicates that patients may become embarrassed when discussing their genitals so it is important to try to put them at ease (Bickley 2016, Collins-Bride and Saxe 2013; Dains et al. 2012, 2015). It is essential that the sexual history and examination should be undertaken in a sensitive manner. Reassure the patient that the information shared will remain confidential. This will help encourage the patient to be more open and honest with you. Take time and give clear explanations as to why you are asking certain questions. If you use careful questioning and tact, patients are more likely to provide you with answers that will assist in reaching a diagnosis. It is useful to begin by stating something like 'I am now going to ask you some questions about your sexual health and practices'. Try to determine the patient's risk of acquiring a sexually transmitted

Pocket Guide to Physical Assessment, First Edition. Edited by Carol Lynn Cox.

infection (STI). Depending on the problem you may wish to begin by asking general questions about sexual function, sexual history, duration of their relationships, and timing of their last sexual encounter.

Questions to ask are:

- whether the patient's sexual relationship is with a regular or casual partner
- the contraceptive methods used
- the number of sexual partners that they have had
- their sexual orientation.
- having sex with men and women or both
- whether their partner has any symptoms
- any previous STIs and any previous treatments
- previously had an STI and symptoms he had
- previous sexual health check-ups
- the use of injected drugs
- any vaccinations against hepatitis A or B
- have been tested for HIV, hepatitis, or syphilis (Ball et al. 2014a, b; Bickley and Szilagyi 2013; Dains et al. 2012, 2015; Japp and Robertson 2013; Jarvis 2015; Rhoads and Paterson 2013).

7.2 General Examination

7.2.1 Important Symptoms to Consider

- urethral discharge
- warts
- ulceration
- testicular pain
- swelling
- ulceration
- rashes
- inflammation
- frequency and urgency
- hesitancy

- haematuria
- nocturia
- impotence
- loss of sexual desire
- infertility
- incontinence
- oliguria
- dysuria (Bickley and Szilagyi 2013; Dains et al. 2012, 2015; Seidel et al. 2010, Swartz 2014; Talley and O'Connor 2014)

7.2.2 Erectile Function

If the presenting problem is erectile dysfunction (ED) ask the following questions:

- Are you suffering from stress – in work or relationships?
- Are you afraid that sexual intercourse may cause cardiac problems?
- Do you drink alcohol? How much? How often?
- What medications do you take? Over the counter? Prescription and/or illicit drugs?
- Do you smoke? How much (number of cigarettes/packs per day)? How often? (Smoking, like alcohol, is a risk factor for ED.)

Note the distribution and amount of body hair, note size of testes as testosterone levels may be reduced.

7.2.3 Possible STI

- To assess the possibility of an STI, ask questions about any discharge or dripping from the penis.
- If the patient has a penile discharge try to ascertain the amount, colour, and consistency.
- Ask if they have any other symptoms such as a temperature, rash, or pain.

- Tell the patient that STIs can affect any opening that comes into contact with sexual organs.
- Ask the patient about oral sex and anal sex and if he answers yes ask about the presence of sore throats, rectal bleeding, pain, itching, or diarrhoea.
- Ask about the presence of any sores, warts, swelling on the penis, or swelling in the scrotum/testicles.
- Ask if the patient has any concerns about HIV infection (Bickley and Szilagyi 2013; Dains et al. 2012, 2015; Japp and Robertson 2013; Jarvis 2015; Tallia and Scherger 2013).

7.2.4 Examination of the Male Genitalia

The patient may lay down or you can ask him to stand whilst you carry out your inspection. Ask in a sensitive way before you proceed, e.g. 'I need to briefly examine you down below. Is that all right?' Then begin your examination by inspecting the penis and groin area. Some examiners recommend that the patient hold his penis during inspection rather than the examiner holding it.

7.3 Inspection

- Note the size, colour, shape, and the presence or absence of a prepuce (foreskin). The size of the penis is usually dependent on the patient's age and overall development.
- Note any abnormal curvatures.
- Examine penis – retract the prepuce (foreskin) to expose glans – it may be useful to get the patient to do this for you. Note the presence of any chancres, ulceration, or erythema and the presence of smegma, which is a cheesy white substance that accumulates normally under the foreskin.

- Examine and inspect the glans; look for the presence of warts, ulcers, nodules, or the signs of any inflammation. Examine the external urethral meatus. If you are a female examiner, ask the patient to squeeze it open gently in an anterior–posterior direction to open the external urethral meatus to inspect for discharge (normally you will find none). If you are a male examiner you will find it easier to do this yourself unless the patient expresses concerns about you doing this.
- Balanitis (inflamed glans of penis) should remind the examiner to check for diabetes.
- If any discharge is noted, take a swab and send it for microbiology examination.
- Inspect the skin around the groin for any excoriation or inflammation. Note the presence of any nits or lice – these can usually be found at the base of the pubic hairs.
- Lift up the scrotum to inspect the posterior surface.
- Note any obvious hernia.
- Examine scrotal swellings – transilluminate (use a torch or flashlight) to discern the presence of fluid.
- A poorly developed scrotum on one or both sides may suggest cryptorchidism (Cox 2010; Swartz 2014; Talley and O'Connor 2014).

7.3.1 Abnormalities of the Penis

- priapism (persistent, usually painful, erection of the penis)
- hypospadias or epispadias (birth defects where the urethra and urethral groove are malformed)
- phimosis (tight prepuce that cannot be retracted over the glans). Note that this is normal in babies
- paraphimosis (a tight prepuce that once retracted cannot be returned and oedema may occur) is common

following the insertion of a catheter and the healthcare professional does not return the prepuce over the glans (Bickley and Szilagyi 2013; Dains et al. 2012, 2015; Japp and Robertson 2013; Jarvis 2015; Rundio 2017; Seidel et al. 2010; Swartz 2014; Talley and O'Connor 2014).

7.3.2 Abnormalities of the Scrotum

- cryptorchidism (undescended testis)
- inguinal hernia
- cystic swelling
- variocele (Occurs in about 8% of male population. It will feel like a bag of worms). Occurs because of varicosity of the veins of the pampiniform plexus.
- epididymal cyst
- hydrocele
- scrotal swelling (common scrotal swellings include inguinal hernias, scrotal oedema, and hydroceles). Tender painful swellings may indicate acute orchitis, acute epididymitis, and torsion of the spermatic cord. Swelling in the scrotum can be evaluated by transillumination (Bickley and Szilagyi 2013; Dains et al. 2012, 2015; Japp and Robertson 2013; Jarvis 2015; Rundio 2017; Seidel et al. 2010; Swartz 2014; Talley and O'Connor 2014).

7.3.3 Look for Signs of Syphilis – Primary, Secondary, and Tertiary

- chancre (painless hard ulcer with a clearly defined rim/edge) seen in primary syphilis
- skin rash, with brown sores about the size of a penny, the rash may cover the whole body or appear only in a few areas. It is almost always on the palms of the hands and soles of the feet and may be seen in secondary syphilis.

- mild pyrexia, fatigue, headache, sore throat, patchy hair loss, and swollen lymph glands throughout the body. These symptoms may be very mild and, like the chancre of primary syphilis, will disappear without treatment.
- In tertiary syphilis, the brain, nervous system, heart, eyes, bones, joints can be affected. This stage can last for years and may result in mental illness, blindness, other neurological problems, heart disease, and death (Bickley and Szilagyi 2013; Dains et al. 2012, 2015; Japp and Robertson 2013; Jarvis 2015; Seidel et al. 2010; Swartz 2014; Talley and O'Connor 2014).

7.3.4 Look for Signs of Gonorrhoea

- painful urination
- yellowish urethral discharge
- painful discharge of bloody pus from the rectum (rectal gonorrhoea)
- throat infection can occur as a result of oral sex with infected partner
  (Note that disseminated gonorrhoea can cause purulent arthritis – often of the knee joint.)

7.3.5 Look for Signs of Herpes

- painful blisters or bumps in the genital or rectal area that crust over, form a scab, and heal
- patient complains of itching, burning, or tingling sensation in the genitals
- inguinal lymphadenopathy (swollen, tender lymph nodes)
- headache
- muscle ache
- pyrexia
- penis discharge

- infection of the urethra causing a burning sensation
- during urination (Bickley and Szilagyi 2013; Dains et al. 2012, 2015; Japp and Robertson 2013; Jarvis 2015; Rundio 2017; Seidel et al. 2010; Swartz 2014; Talley and O'Connor 2014).

7.3.6 Look for Signs of Human Papilloma Virus (HPV) Infection

- genital warts (condylomata acuminata) usually appear as small bumps or groups of bumps. They can be raised or flat, single or multiple, small or large, and sometimes cauliflower shaped.

7.3.7 Look for Signs of Chlamydia

- no symptoms in 70–80% of cases
- lower abdominal pain and burning pain during urination
- mucopurulent discharge from the penis
- tenderness or pain in the testicles
- burning and itching around the meatus
- rectal pain, discharge, or bleeding in patients who engage in anal sex

7.4 Palpation

7.4.1 Groin

- The spermatic cord, lymph nodes, and arteries occupy the groin.
- Swellings here are usually caused by hernias or enlarged lymph nodes.
- Palpate the groin to detect enlarged lymph nodes.
- Most people have small, shotty nodes. Most enlarged tender nodes arise from infection in the legs or feet. However, in some Afro-Caribbean men this is normal.

- If large nodes, palpate spleen carefully (*reticulosis* or *leukaemia*) (Bickley and Szilagyi 2013; Dains et al. 2012, 2015; Japp and Robertson 2013; Jarvis 2015; Rundio 2017; Seidel et al. 2010; Swartz 2014; Talley and O'Connor 2014).

7.4.2 Hernia

When checking for the presence of hernia examine the patient standing and ask him to cough – enlargement of a groin swelling suggests a hernia.

- indirect (oblique) inguinal hernia: swelling reduced to internal inguinal ring by pressure on contents of hernial sac and then controlled by pressure over the internal ring when patient asked to cough; if your hand is then removed, impulse passes medially towards external ring and is palpable above the pubic tubercle
- direct inguinal hernia: impulse in a forward direction mainly above groin crease medial to femoral artery and swelling not controlled by pressure over internal ring
- femoral hernia: swelling fills out the groin crease medial to the femoral artery (Bickley and Szilagyi 2013; Dains et al. 2012, 2015; Japp and Robertson 2013; Jarvis 2015; Rundio 2017; Seidel et al. 2010; Swartz 2014; Talley and O'Connor 2014).

7.4.3 Penis

Palpate the whole length of the penis to the perineum and note the state of the dorsal vein. Note any hardened or tender areas. Hardness may indicate a urethral stricture or cancer whereas tenderness may indicate an infection.

7.4.4 Scrotum

- Ask 'Is your scrotum painful anywhere? Tell me if I hurt you'.
- Warm your hands and remember to use gentle pressure.
- Palpate the scrotum for the testes and epididymis.
- Palpate each testes and epididymis with your thumb and first 2 fingers.
- Observe the patients face.
- *Note the size, shape, and consistency of each testis. Note any tenderness.*
- Tender and enlarged testes may occur with *orchitis* or *torsion of the testis. Multiple torturous veins may indicate a variocele.*
- A large, soft swelling which transilluminates suggests *hydrocele* or an *epididymal cyst*. A hydrocele surrounds the testis; an epididymal cyst lies behind the testis.
- A large, hard, painless testis suggests testicular cancer, a potentially curable cancer with a peak incidence between the ages of 15 and 35 years.

7.4.5 Prostate Gland

- Lay the patient on the left side with knees flexed to the chest or if he can, ask the patient to bend over the examination table.
- Inspect anus for lumps, haemorrhoids, fissures, ulcers, inflammation, excoriation, and warts.
    - *Explain to the patient that you will need to place your finger into his rectum to examine the prostate. This procedure may be uncomfortable but should not be painful.* Say: 'I am going to put a finger into your back passage'.
- With lubricant on glove, press your fingertip against the anal verge then gently slip forefinger into anal

canal and then into the rectum. Inform the patient that he may feel the urge to pass urine but he will not. It helps to have the patient push whilst you insert your finger. Palpate the prostate gland on the anterior rectal wall. Check the size and character of the prostate. It should feel smooth and rubbery and be approximately the size of a walnut. Note any nodules or tenderness. A swollen tender prostate may indicate acute prostatitis whereas an enlarged smooth but firm prostate may indicate benign prostatic hypertrophy. Hard roughened areas are suggestive of cancer.

References

Ball, J., Dains, J., Flynn, J. et al. (2014a). *Seidel's Guide to Physical Examination*, 8e. St. Louis: Mosby.

Ball, J., Dains, J., Flynn, J. et al. (2014b). *Student Laboratory Manual to Accompany Seidel's Guide to Physical Examination*, 8e. St. Louis: Mosby.

Bickley, L. and Szilagyi, P. (2013). *Bates' Guide to Physical Examination and History Taking*, 11e. New York: Wolters Kluwer/Lippincott Williams & Wilkins.

Bickley, L. S. (2016). Male genitalia and hernias. In: *Bates Pocket Guide to Physical Examination and History Taking*, 12e, 541–564. Philadelphia, London: Wolters Kluwer/Lippincott Williams & Wilkins

Collins-Bride, G. and Saxe, J. (2013). *Clinical Guidelines for Advanced Practice Nursing – An Interdisciplinary Approach*, 2e. Burlington, MA: Jones and Bartlett Learning.

Cox, C. (2010). *Physical Assessment for Nurses*, 2e. Oxford: Wiley Blackwell.

Dains, J., Baumann, L., and Scheibel, P. (2012). *Advanced Health Assessment and Clinical Diagnosis in Primary Care*, 4e. St. Louis: Elsevier.

Dains, J., Baumann, L., and Scheibel, P. (2015). *Advanced Health Assessment and Clinical Diagnosis in Primary Care*, 5e. St. Louis: Mosby.

Japp, A. and Robertson, C. (2013). *Macleod's Clinical Diagnosis*. Edinburgh: Churchill Livingstone, Elsevier.

Jarvis, C. (2015). *Physical Examination and Health Assessment*, 7e. Edinburgh: Elsevier.

Rhoads, J. and Paterson (2013). *Advanced Health Assessment and Diagnostic Reasoning*, 2e. Burlington: Jones and Bartlett.

Rundio, A. (2017). Men's health. In: *Lippincott Certification Review: Family Nurse Practitioner & Adult-Gerontology Nurse Practitioner* (ed. A. Rundio and W. Lorman), 224–238. New York: Wolters Kluwer.

Seidel, H., Ball, J., Dains, J., and Benedict, G. (2010). *Mosby's Physical Examination Handbook*, 7e. St. Louis: Mosby-Year Book.

Swartz, M. (2014). *Physical Diagnosis: History and Examination*, With Student Consult Online Access, 7e. London: Elsevier.

Talley, N. and O'Connor, S. (2014). *Clinical Examination: A Systematic Guide to Physical Diagnosis*, 7e. London: Churchill Livingstone, Elsevier.

Tallia, A. and Scherger, J. (2013). *Swanson's Family Practice Review*, 6e. St. Louis: Mosby.

8 Examination of the Female Genitalia

Victoria Lack[1,2]

[1] Department of Health Sciences, University of York, York, UK

[2] Beech House Surgery, Knaresborough, North Yorkshire, UK

8.1 General Examination

This chapter addresses examination of a nonpregnant adult female. Examination of a woman's reproductive system includes an abdominal examination (refer to Chapter 6), examination of the external genitalia, a speculum examination, and bimanual examination. A rectal examination may also be needed in some circumstances. Examination of the inguinal lymph nodes should also be performed. You should not proceed with an examination if you think the woman is not able to cope with the procedure; e.g. if the client is unduly stressed or upset, has had previous vasovagal reactions, or has an imperforate hymen (RCN 2013). You should also not proceed with the examination unless you are fully knowledgeable of the anatomy and physiology of the female reproductive system.

The following considers the pelvic examination of a nonpregnant woman.

The examination is regarded by women as extremely intimate. It is a procedure that most women in western

Pocket Guide to Physical Assessment, First Edition. Edited by Carol Lynn Cox.

cultures will experience at some point in their lives. It is your responsibility to make the examination as bearable as possible. Some, but not all women will prefer a female examiner to carry out the examination. This wish should be respected. In emergency situations, where it is not practicable to delay the examination, if a female examiner is not available, sensible and practicable measures must be taken (RCN 2013). All women should be offered a chaperone, regardless of the gender of the person carrying out the examination. This is not only to protect the patient but also to protect the clinician. Some women may want to have a friend or relative present. It is important for you as the examiner undertaking the procedure to establish a rapport with the woman prior to examination. It is also important that you explain fully the procedure and why it is necessary, prior to the woman getting undressed and exposed. A diagram or model may help here. However, it is equally important to be aware that some women do not want to have a detailed explanation and would rather you 'just got on with it'.

This chapter does not address the physical examination of a female child, which should be carried out only by specialist staff but does present issues associated with examination of the child. Equally, you must assess the capacity of adults to decide if they are fully concordant with the examination prior to procedure. If there is an indication that a child or young person has been sexually abused, you should follow local guidelines and refer immediately.

8.2 Preparation

Ask the woman if she needs to empty her bladder prior to the examination. Make sure everything is ready before asking the woman to get undressed. Ensure there is a good lighting source, like the Welch Allen speculum light for use with disposable specula, or other source that can be positioned to give the best view of the genitalia. Check the light before the examination to ensure it works. Secure the door to the consultation room and let the woman know that the door is closed and no one else will come in. Explain exactly what you want the woman to do. It may seem evident that you need the woman to remove her underwear, but it may not be evident to the woman. Leave the woman to undress in private, having given her a gown or blanket or paper drape to put over herself so she is not sitting exposed.

In most primary care settings, the woman will be asked to lie on a couch/table in the dorsal position, with her feet either in stirrups or the soles of her feet together and knees apart. In secondary care, the lithotomy position – using leg supports – is more common. The lithotomy position gives a better view of the genitalia. A left lateral position may also be used, which is useful in examining women who have utero-vaginal prolapse or vesicovaginal fistulae (Arulkamaran et al. 2007). In this case a Sims speculum should be used. This position may also be a more comfortable position for older women, particularly if they have kyphosis or arthritis/bone/joint disease. Once the woman is in the correct position, covered over her abdomen and legs with a gown or drape, check again that everything is at hand. Always wash your hands and then put on gloves (Table 8.1).

A complete examination of the female genitalia consists of the following components:

- external genitalia – inspection
- external genitalia – palpation
- speculum examination
- bimanual ('per vagina' or 'PV' examination)
(Thomas and Monaghan 2010).

Table 8.1 Materials needed for a pelvic examination.

Gloves (check size prior to gloves)
Warm water for lubrication
Water-based lubrication jelly
Specula (It may be necessary to use different sizes to ensure comfort and facilitate visualisation of the cervix.). As a general rule short obese women will require a short wide speculum; medium-sized women will require a medium-/regular-sized speculum. Tall thin women will require a medium-/regular-sized speculum or a long thin speculum. A multipara woman (five vaginal deliveries or more) will require a large speculum to keep the vaginal walls from falling in and obscuring your view. Nulliparous women will require a small speculum. An older postmenopausal female may require a small or paediatric speculum. A female child will require a paediatric speculum.
Cervical broom and brush (Note the brush is not normally used.)
Liquid-based cytology (LBC) container (if cervical cytology is being undertaken.)
Cotton tip applicator (to remove heavy secretions obscuring the cervical os)
Sterile swabs and correct microbial/viral specimen tube (if samples are being taken for microbiology/virology)
Slides with covers (for microscopy on site)
Culture tube with swabs (for suspected chlamydia or gonorrhoea). Note that in some laboratories, a clean catch urine is preferred for laboratory determination of chlamydia/gonorrhoea.
pH paper (for testing the pH of the vagina)
Light source (Welch Allen specula light or goose neck lamp)
Haemocult test kit (when performing a rectal examination) for occult blood
Tissues/feminine hygiene wipes

8.3 Inspection of the External Genitalia

Tell the woman you are beginning the examination. Look at the perineum. Note hygiene and distribution of pubic hair. Look at the labia majora, which should be generally symmetrical but may be open or closed, full or thin. Note any lesions. Open the labia majora to inspect the labia minora, which should be darker coloured and soft. Inspect the clitoris, urethral meatus, and vaginal opening. Check for any inflammation, redness or discharge, ulceration, bruises and atrophy. Ask the patient to 'bear down' and/or to cough to look at the vaginal walls to check for any prolapse.

Palpate the labia majora, which should be pliant and fleshy with the index finger and thumb. Palpate for the Bartholin glands, which are located in the posterolateral labia majora. These will be palpable only if the duct becomes obstructed resulting in a painless lump or acute abscess (Jarvis 2015; Thomas and Monaghan 2010).

Palpate the lateral tissue of the perineum between thumb and forefinger. Check for swelling, tenderness, and masses.

8.4 Speculum Examination (Figure 8.1)

A speculum examination is carried out to see further into the vagina, visualise the cervix, take high vaginal and endocervical swabs, and perform cervical cytology. The bivalve Cusco's (disposable) speculum is the most commonly used. Metal bivalve specula, which are reusable following sterilisation, are preferred by some clinicians. Ensure you are familiar with how to open and close the

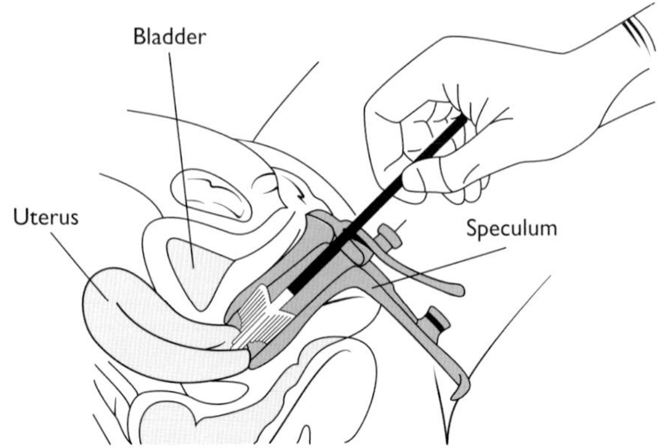

Figure 8.1 Speculum examination. Source: Cox 2009. Reproduced with permission from John Wiley and Sons.

blades. Warm and lubricate the speculum using warm water. Lubricating gel that is water-based can be used as speculum examination is often uncomfortable for women. If a sample for cervical cytology is to be taken use the water-based lubricant only and avoid putting it over the tips of the blades, so as to not contaminate the sample (NHS Cancer Screening Programme 2006). Tell the woman what you are going to do. Place the back of your hand on the woman's inner thigh before touching the labia. This will help to alleviate the startle effect prior to touching the labia. Then gently part the labia to insert the speculum. In the dorsal position the speculum should be inserted with the handle superior, whereas in the lithotomy position the handle is usually inferior (Arulkamaran et al. 2007). You may choose to insert the speculum sideways and rotate the handle into either the superior or inferior position. Using this insertion technique is more comfortable for women. If the handle is superior, make sure that it does not touch the clitoris, which is very sensitive. Insert the speculum in a slightly downwards direction. Check the woman's comfort at this point. Open the speculum when it is fully inserted and flush with the perineum. It may not be necessary to fully open the speculum. Inspect the vaginal walls, which should be pink and moist. The cervix should be visible between the tips of the blades. If you cannot see the cervix try withdrawing the speculum slightly. The cervix may 'drop' into view or you may need to close the speculum, withdraw further, and change direction of the speculum slightly. A digital examination can be used to establish the position of the cervix prior to insertion of the speculum. Putting a pillow under the woman's buttocks or asking her to put her hands underneath her buttocks may also help to better position the woman in order to visualise the cervix (Jarvis 2015).

Inspect the cervix. It should be symmetrical, pink, and about 3 cm in diameter. The cervix should extend approximately 2 cm into the vagina. More than 3 cm could indicate a vaginal prolapse (Jarvis 2015; RCN 2013). The surface of the cervix should be smooth. The cervix is the point where vaginal squamous epithelium meets the endocervical columnar epithelium at the squamocolumnar junction. The level of the junction varies throughout a woman's life and can give a very different appearance to the cervix. An extension of the endocervical epithelium onto the surface of the cervix is often called an 'ectropion' (sometimes called cervical erosion). This is often present at puberty, during pregnancy, and if a woman is taking oestrogen containing hormonal contraception. The os should be round in a nulliparous woman and slitlike (may look like a smile) in a parous woman. There may be some clear or creamy odourless discharge from the os. Note any secretions, polyps, or other lesions. Note any nabothian cysts or follicles. These are normal findings and have the appearance of small yellow nodules (RCN 2013). In pregnancy the cervix may appear different and have a bluish or purple hue (Chadwick sign). The cervix can also change position and look different according to the time of the menstrual cycle as well as pre- and postmenopausally. Cervicitis causes a red and inflamed cervix which bleeds on contact.

Obtain cervical cytological samples and/or swabs at this point as needed. Note any contact bleeding during taking of the samples. This may not necessarily be abnormal; an enthusiastically taken cervical cytology specimen may cause contact bleeding, especially if the patient has an ectropion. Inform the woman that is not uncommon for her to experience some light bleeding post the examination. Remove the speculum with as much care as during insertion. Continue to examine the vaginal walls as the speculum is withdrawn, keeping the blades open until they are clear of the cervix to avoid causing pain. Rotate the speculum a quarter turn so the anterior and posterior walls of the speculum can be examined. Close the blades when they are visible near the introitus. Take care not to pinch the labia or hairs.

8.4.1 Taking a Cervical Sample for Cytology

It makes sense to perform cervical cytology, if it is due, during a speculum examination if the woman is not in distress. It is outside the scope of this chapter to discuss fully cervical cytology. You should ensure you are fully trained according to national and local protocols and are competent to carry out the procedure before doing so. In the United Kingdom and United States of America (USA), liquid-based cytology (**LBC**) is used to perform cervical screening for all women aged 25–64 years every 3 years (up to age 50) and every 5 years (aged over 50) (NHS Choices 2015a). It should be remembered that cervical cytology in primary care is a screening test and should not be used for diagnosis. Of note now human papilloma virus (**HPV**) screening is carried out in conjunction with cervical cytology in the laboratory. There is no difference in how the sample is obtained.

8.4.2 Taking Swabs

Swabs should be taken during a speculum examination if there is concern around infection and/or if there is increased and/or abnormal discharge discussed during history taking and/or found on speculum examination. Swabs should also be taken if the patient is unwell or complaining of abdominal pain. pH paper can also be used to test any vaginal discharge. A normal pH is <4.5.

8.5 Bimanual Examination

The purpose of a bimanual examination is to bring the pelvic organs closer to the abdominal wall, where they can be felt by the hand on the abdomen (Arulkamaran et al. 2007). Explain again to the woman what you are going to do. Using lubrication on gloved fingers, place the index and middle finger of the right or left hand into the vagina, palm upwards (Figure 8.2). One finger can be used if

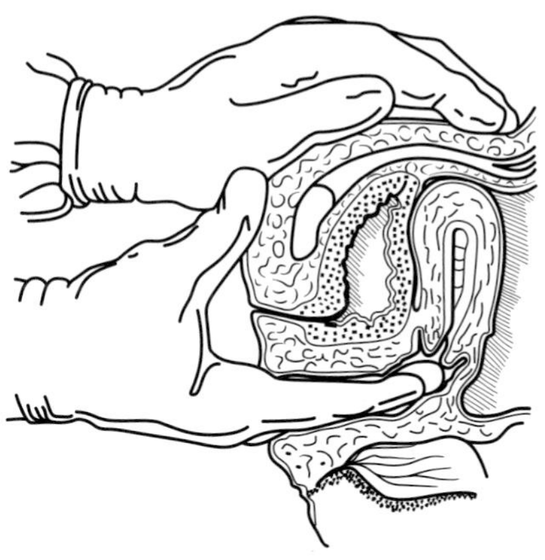

Figure 8.2 Bimanual examination. Source: Cox 2009. Reproduced with permission from John Wiley and Sons.

the woman is anxious or experiences discomfort. Note vaginal wall tone, any prolapse, tenderness, or protrusions. Locate the cervix. The cervix should feel smooth and firm. Check for 'cervical excitation' or 'cervical motion tenderness' by gently pushing the cervix to one side and then the other. This is the equivalent of rebound tenderness in an abdominal examination. Pushing the cervix laterally will stretch the adnexa on the same side of the pelvis. The cervix should move 1–2 cm in either direction without pain. If the procedure elicits pain, this could be because of bleeding from an ectopic pregnancy or inflammation in the adnexa (Cruickshank and Shetty 2009; Jarvis 2015).

8.5.1 Palpate the Uterus

Place the left or right hand over the lower abdomen. Feel the uterus between the hands. An anteverted uterus should be easy to feel. A retroverted one may not be. However, the body of the uterus may be palpable by the vaginal fingers by moving them to above and below the cervix and exerting pressure inwards. The uterus should be pear shaped, about 5.5–8 cm long in nulliparous women, larger in multiparous women (Seidel et al. 2010). The contour should be round, firm, and smooth. The uterus should be slightly mobile in anterior–posterior plane and nontender on movement. Note the presence of any masses.

Next palpate the adnexa by moving the abdominal hand laterally over the lower abdominal quadrant on the same side as the internal fingers, which should be in the lateral fornix of the vagina. Apply firm pressure starting medially to the anterior iliac crest. Note any tenderness or masses. Palpate for the fallopian tubes on either side of the uterus; they should not normally be palpable or the area tender.

Try to palpate the ovaries; this can cause discomfort in women. The ovaries are 2–4 cm long, about the size of an almond. They are sensitive to touch but should not be acutely tender. They should be smooth, firm, and mobile. In postmenopausal women they are smaller and should not be palpable. Finally, place the vaginal fingers in the posterior fornix with the abdominal hand pressing down over the abdomen. The pouch of Douglas and uterosacral ligaments may then be felt. Note any tenderness and nodularity of the ligaments.

Having finished the examination, offer the woman some tissues/feminine wipes and sanitary pads if needed and leave her to dress in private. Ensure she is able to wash her hands.

8.6 Documentation

The following points should be included in the records (Jarvis 2015; RCN 2013):

- external genitalia
- vagina
- cervix
- uterus
- adnexa.

They may include reference to:

- size
- position
- consistency
- mobility
- mass
- tenderness.

Provide correct information about the findings and results of the examination. If swabs have been taken or screening performed this should also be included.

8.7 Female Genital Mutilation

With any discussion concerning examination of the female reproductive system, it is necessary to note the possibility of female genital mutilation (**FGM**). This is defined as procedures which intentionally alter or cause injury to the genital organs for nonmedical reasons. There are four main types of FGM:

- **Type 1 – clitoridectomy** – removing part of or the entire clitoris.
- **Type 2 – excision** – removing part or all of the clitoris and the inner labia (lips that surround the vagina), with or without removal of the labia majora (larger outer lips).
- **Type 3 – infibulation** – narrowing of the vaginal opening by creating a seal, formed by cutting and repositioning the labia.
- **Other harmful procedures** to the female genitals, which include pricking, piercing, cutting, scraping, and burning the area (NHS Choices 2015a).

FGM is illegal in the United Kingdom and the United States of America (The Guardian 2014; 18 U.S. Code § 116 1996). In all cases if you are worried about a child under 18 who is at risk of FGM or has had FGM, you have a legal obligation to share this information with social care and the police. It is then their responsibility to investigate, safeguard, and protect any girls involved. Other professionals should not attempt to investigate cases themselves. However, it is important to note that as with domestic violence and rape, if an adult woman has had FGM and this is identified through the delivery of healthcare, the patient's right to patient confidentiality MUST be respected if they do not wish any action to be taken. No reports to social services or the police should be made in these cases. For detailed guidance for clinicians who encounter FGM please refer to the guidelines available via NHS Choices 2015b; USAID.GOV 2016).

For women who have undergone FGM, examination may be psychologically difficult and physically painful or impossible. All women who have had FGM should be offered referral to specialist services.

8.8 Overview of Common Presentations

Examples of common presentations:

- abnormal bleeding
- vulval symptoms
- vaginal discharge
- genital prolapse
- pelvic pain including dyspareunia
- pelvic masses
- abnormal bleeding from the vagina

Remember to exclude pregnancy first. Non-pregnancy related causes of abnormal bleeding patterns can be classified as:

- intermenstrual bleeding (**IMB**)
- postcoital bleeding (**PCB**)
- breakthrough bleeding (**BTB**)
- postmenopausal bleeding (**PMB**)
- menorrhagia
- amenorrhoea.

Causes of some abnormal bleeding patterns:

IMB	PCB	BTB
Pregnancy related (including ectopic and molar pregnancy)	Cervical ectropian	Combined oral contraceptive pill
Physiological; around ovulation (spotting) and perimenopausal (diagnosis of exclusion)	Cervical or endo-metrial polyps	Pre or post
Vaginal cancer	Vaginal cancer	Depot injection
Vaginitis (rare prior to menopause)	Cervical cancer	Intrauterine system
Sexually trans-mitted infections (STIs) gonorrhoea, chlamydia, and less commonly trichomoniasis vaginalis)	Trauma	Emergency hormonal contraception
Cervical polyps/warts/ ectropion/cancer	No specific cause found in approximately 50% of women	
Uterine fibroids		
Uterine cancer		
Oestrogen secreting ovarian tumours		
Iatrogenic (certain drugs, missed pills/following treatment to the cervix)		

Source: Adapted from (Patient 2015a).

The important point is first to rule out pregnancy and second to be aware of the risk of female cancers. In the United Kingdom (UK), refer to the National Institute for Health and Care Excellence (**NICE**) national guidelines for suspected cancer (NICE 2017). In the United States (USA), refer to the American Cancer Society guidelines for screening/suspected cancer (ACS 2014). Vaginal bleeding after the menopause is a worrying sign. An urgent referral is recommended for women who have PMB. It needs prompt investigation as it could indicate malignancy. The 2017 UK cancer guidelines state that women should be referred using a suspected cancer pathway referral for an appointment within two weeks for suspected endometrial cancer if they are aged 55 and over with PMB (unexplained vaginal bleeding more than 12 months after menstruation has stopped because of the menopause). Consider a suspected cancer pathway referral (for an appointment within two weeks) for endometrial cancer in women aged under 55 with PMB (NICE 2017). Similar rules apply in USA.

8.8.1 Menorrhagia

Menorraghia is defined as > 80 ml of blood loss per period (normal is 20–60 ml) (Thomas and Monaghan 2010). In practice, this is difficult to measure. Some causes of menorrhagia are listed here:

- hypothyroidism
- copper intrauterine device (**IUD**)
- fibroids
- endometriosis
- polyps of the cervix or uterus
- sexually transmitted infections (**STIs**)
- previous sterilisation
- drugs (warfarin/aspirin/nonsteroidal anti-inflammatory drugs)
- clotting disorders (Thomas and Monaghan 2010).

8.8.2 Amenorrhea

Can be primary (failure to menstruate by age 16) or secondary where there is a history of normal menarche, then no menses for six months (Thomas and Monaghan 2010). It is necessary first to exclude pregnancy, and then further investigations are necessary to determine the cause, which could be endocrine, local ovarian causes, or physical or emotional stress.

8.8.3 Vulval Signs and Symptoms

Conditions affecting the vulva include:

- infection (candida, genital herpes, genital warts)
- vulval dystrophy
- dermatological disorders (lichen planus)
- cancer.

Candida usually presents with itching and burning of vulva and/or the vaginal walls, alongside a 'cottage cheese' looking vaginal discharge. With genital herpes there are usually bilateral crops of vesicles or ulcers on the vulva and sometimes the vagina and cervix. There may also be local oedema of the labia and vaginal discharge. The inguinal lymph nodes will usually be enlarged (Patient 2015b). Genital warts usually present as painless crops of lesions. They may be skin coloured, red, white, grey, or brown and may be broad based or pedunculated. They usually appear fleshy and soft in nonhairy areas but firmer in areas with pubic hair. They may appear on labia, clitoris, urethral meatus, introitus, vagina, and cervix as well as the anus. Visible genital warts are transmitted by the HPV virus but have a low risk of malignancy. They can be associated with increased vaginal discharge, PMB, and IMB. They can also be associated with other STIs. Referral to a sexual health clinic is usually indicated (Patient 2015b).

Vulval dystrophy and atrophic vaginitis are caused by a lack of oestrogen, e.g. in postmenopausal women. The labia appear thin, pale, and dry as will the vaginal walls. It can also cause superficial dyspareunia, minor vaginal bleeding, and pain (Thomas and Monaghan 2010).

Almost any skin condition can affect the vulva. Dermatitis can appear as a red rash or area of inflammation of the labia and introitus. It is often secondary to application of products sold for cleansing of the genital area or irritation secondary to urinary incontinence. Lichen planus presents with intense redness and oedema of the vulva and superficial ulceration. It can lead to scarring and narrowing of the introitus over time if not treated, resembling chronic lichen sclerosis. This condition can present with vulval lesions leading to a 'cigarette' paper appearance – thin, white, and crinkly skin. Again, the introitus will shrink and the labia minora may become fused together. Treatment is usually with potent topical steroids (Patient 2015b).

8.8.4 Cancer of the Vulva/Vagina

A lump may be present or ulcer which may be associated with bleeding. Associated symptoms may be itching and pain. The 2014 ACS and the 2015 UK cancer guidelines recommend the following:

8.8.4.1 Vulval Cancer

- Consider a suspected cancer pathway referral (for an appointment within two weeks) for vulval cancer in women with an unexplained vulval lump, ulceration, or bleeding.

8.8.4.2 Vaginal Cancer

- Consider a suspected cancer pathway referral (for an appointment within two weeks) for vaginal cancer in women with an unexplained palpable mass in or at the entrance to the vagina.

8.8.5 Vaginal Discharge

Symptoms suggesting that discharge is abnormal include:

- a discharge that is heavier than usual
- a discharge that is thicker than usual
- puslike discharge
- white and clumpy discharge
- greyish, greenish, yellowish, or blood-tinged discharge
- foul-smelling (fishy or rotting meat) discharge
- a discharge accompanied by bloodiness, itching, burning, rash, or soreness (Patient 2015a).

Discharge can be caused by infection but can also be altered due to noninfective causes such as

- physiological causes; stage in menstrual cycle/ pre- postmenopausal
- cervical polyps and ectopy
- foreign bodies – e.g. retained tampon
- vulval dermatitis
- erosive lichen planus
- genital tract malignancy – e.g. cancer of the cervix, uterus, or ovary
- fistulae.

8.8.5.1 Nonsexually Transmitted

Vulvovaginal candida has been discussed previously and usually produces a thick white discharge which is slightly lumpy and may have a 'cottage cheese' like appearance. There is usually no odour. Bacterial vaginosis usually causes a thin profuse fishy smelling discharge.

8.8.5.2 Sexually Transmitted

Trichomonas vaginalis may cause a thick, profuse yellowy discharge which may be frothy with an offensive odour. Chlamydia may produce a profuse vaginal discharge, but it is important to remember that the infection is asymptomatic in 80% of women. Gonorrhoea may present with a profuse discharge but again is asymptomatic in up to 50% women (Patient 2015c).

Swabs should be taken, using the correct swab for each procedure according to national and local guidelines. It is acceptable if the woman prefers take her own vaginal swabs.

Normal practice in the UK and USA is to take two or three swabs as below. The swabs used are:

- high vaginal swab in transport medium to diagnose vaginal infections and bacterial vaginosis
- endocervical swab in transport medium to diagnose gonorrhoea
- endocervical swab for a chlamydial nucleic acid amplification test (**NAAT**) to diagnose chlamydia.

However, current guidelines suggest if a simple, non sexually transmitted infection is suspected, then high vaginal swabs are needed only if there is treatment failure, in pregnancy, postpartum, posttermination, or postsurgical procedures (RCGP and BASHH 2013).

8.8.6 Genital Prolapse

Genital prolapse is descent of the pelvic organs through the pelvic floor into the vaginal canal. This includes:

- uterocoele: uterus
- urethrocoele: urethra
- cystocoele: bladder
- enterocoele; small bowel
- rectocoele: rectum

The above will present clinically as a bulge in the vaginal wall, either anteriorly (in the case of bladder and or urethral prolapse), apically (uterine prolapse), or posteriorly (rectal prolapse). The degree of uterine descent in a uterine prolapse can be graded by the Baden–Walker or Beecham classification systems:

- first degree: cervix visible when the perineum is depressed – prolapse is contained within the vagina
- second degree: cervix prolapsed through the introitus with the fundus remaining in the pelvis
- third degree: procidentia (complete prolapse) – entire uterus is outside the introitus (Patient 2015d).

Treatment can include pelvic floor exercises, vaginal pessaries, or surgical intervention for severe cases.

8.8.7 Pelvic Pain and Dyspareunia

Distinguishing between pain of gynaecological origin and gastrointestinal origin is difficult as the female reproductive organs share the same innervations for the lower ileum, sigmoid colon, and rectum. Careful history taking and abdominal as well as pelvic examination is needed. As with all pain, it may be acute or chronic in nature. Dyspareunia (pain on sexual intercourse) is often associated with chronic pelvic pain (Table 8.2).

8.8.8 Pelvic Inflammatory Disease

Pelvic inflammatory disease (**PID**) is a syndrome resulting from the spread of microorganisms to the endometrium and fallopian tubes. It is often caused by a variety of organisms and is not necessarily due to STIs (Patient 2015e). History includes high fever, acute pelvic pain and dyspareunia, abnormal vaginal bleeding, and purulent vaginal discharge. On pelvic examination there is cervical motion tenderness and adnexal tenderness (Sadler et al. 2008).

Table 8.2 Differential diagnosis of acute pelvic pain.

Category	Diagnosis
Gynaecological	
Pregnancy related	Ectopic Miscarriage Complications in later pregnancy
Ovarian	Mittelschmerz Torsion/rupture/haemorrhage of an ovarian cyst Ovarian hyperstimulation syndrome
Tubal	Pelvic inflammatory disease (**PID**)
Uterine	Dysmenorrhoea Fibroid degeneration
Pelvic	Endometriosis Tumour
Nongynaecological	
Gastrointestinal	Appendicitis Inflammatory bowel disease Diverticulitis Constipation Adhesions Strangulated hernia
Urinary tract	Infection Calculus Retention

Source: Adapted from O'Connor and Kovacs (2003)

8.8.9 Endometriosis

Endometriosis is the presence of tissue similar to the endometrium found outside of the uterine cavity, most commonly in the pelvis. History includes pelvic pain, dyspareunia, dysmenorrhoea, menorrhagia, and infertility. On examination, there may be pelvic tenderness, pelvic mass, and fixation of the uterus (Sadler et al. 2008).

8.8.10 Fibroids (Uterine Leiomyoma)

Fibroids are benign tumours of the myometrium. Usually they are asymptomatic, but they may cause menorrhagia, pain, pelvic discomfort, and backache as well as urinary symptoms. On examination, the uterus will feel 'bulky' and there may be a pelvic mass (Sadler et al. 2008).

8.8.11 Ovarian Cancer

Ovarian cancer may present with many symptoms, including abdominal and or pelvic pain as well as abdominal distension or 'bloating', early satiety, and loss of appetite. Late symptoms may include ascites and or pelvic or abdominal mass. Refer to current cancer pathway guidelines for urgent referral guidance. ACS (2014) and the 2017 UK cancer guidelines (ACS 2014; NICE 2017)

8.8.12 Pelvic Masses

The main differential diagnoses are outlined in the table below:

Pregnancy

	Example	Nature of mass
Ovarian mass	Benign tumour, functional cysts, ovarian cancer	Painless mass, often one side
Uterine mass	Fibroids	'Bulky' uterus
Tubal mass	Chronic salpingitis	Tender mass

Source: Lewellyn et al. (2014).

As above, all masses should be referred urgently for further investigation unless there is a clear and benign cause.

References

ACS (2014) American Cancer Society Guidelines for the Early Detection of Cancerhttps://www.cancer.org/healthy/find-cancer-early/cancer-screening-guidelines/american-cancer-society-guidelines-for-the-early-detection-of-cancer.html (accessed 26 September 2018)

Arulkamaran, S., Symonds, I., and Fowlie, A. (2007). *Oxford Handbook of Obstetrics and Gynaecology*. New York: Oxford University Press.

Cruickshank, M. and Shetty, A. (2009). *Obstetrics and Gynaecology, Clinical Cases Uncovered*. Oxford: Wiley-Blackwell.

Cox, C.L, (2009). *Physical Assessment for Nurses* (2nd Ed.). Oxford:Wiley-Blackwell.

Jarvis, C. (2015). *Physical Examination and Health Assessment*, 7e. Edinburgh: Elsevier.

Lewellyn, H., Ang, H., Lewis, K., and Al'Abdullah, A. (2014). *Oxford Handbook of Clinical Diagnosis*, 3e. Oxford: Oxford University Press.

NHS Cancer Screening Programme (2006) *Cervical Screening: Professional Guidance*. https://www.gov.uk/government/collections/cervical-screening-professional-guidance (accessed 28 August 2018).

NHS Choices (2015a) *Cervical Screening*. http://www.nhs.uk/Conditions/Cervical-screening-test/Pages/Introduction.aspx (accessed 14 October 2015).

NHS Choices (2015b) *Female Genital Mutilation*. http://www.nhs.uk/conditions/female-genital-mutilation/Pages/Introduction.aspx (accessed 14 October 2015).

NICE (2017) Suspected cancer:recognition and referral. *Suspected Cancer Recognition and Referral Overview*. https://pathways.nice.org.uk/pathways/suspected-cancer-recognition-and-referral.

O'Connor, V. and Kovacs, G. (2003). *Obstetrics, Gynaecology and Women's Health*. Cambridge: Cambridge University Press.

Patient (2015a) *Intermenstrual and Postcoital Bleeding*. http://patient.info/doctor/intermenstrual-and-postcoital-bleeding (accessed 22 August 2015).

Patient (2015b) *Vulval Problems*. http://patient.info/doctor/vulval-problems-pro (accessed 22 August 2015).

Patient (2015c) *Vaginal Discharge*. http://patient.info/doctor/vaginal-discharge (accessed 22 August 2015).

Patient (2015d) *Genitourinary Prolapse*. http://patient.info/doctor/genitourinary-prolapse-pro (accessed 21 September 2015).

Patient (2015e) *Pelvic Inflammatory Disease*. http://patient.info/doctor/pelvic-inflammatory-disease-pro (accessed 21 September 2015).

Royal College of General Practitioners & British Association for Sexual Health and HIV) (2013) *Sexually Transmitted Infections in Primary Care (2nd ed.)* http://www.bashh.org/documents/Sexually%20Transmitted%20Infections%20in%20Primary%20Care%202013.pdf (accessed 21 September 2015).

Royal College of Nursing (2013) *Genital Examination in Women*. www.rcn.org.uk/professional-development/publications/pub-005480 (accessed 28 August 2018).

Sadler, C., White, J., Everitt, H., and Simon, C. (2008). *Women's Health: Oxford General Practice Library*. Oxford: Oxford University Press.

Seidel, H., Ball, J., Dains, J., and Benedict, G. (2010). *Mosby's Physical Examination Handbook*, 7e. St. Louis: Mosby-Year Book.

The Guardian (2014) FGM is banned but very much alive in the UK. https://www.theguardian.com/society/2014/feb/06/female-genital-mutilation-foreign-crime-common-uk (accessed 21 January 2018).

Thomas, J. and Monaghan, T. (2010). *Oxford Handbook of Clinical Examination and Practical Skills*, 2e. Oxford: Oxford University Press.

USAID.GOV (2016) Female genital mutilation/cutting: United States Government's response https://www.usaid.gov/news-information/fact-sheets/female-genital-mutilation-cutting-usg-response (accessed 26 September 2018)

18 U.S. Code § 116 –Female genital mutilation. (1996) *LII / Legal Information Institute*. https://www.law.cornell.edu/uscode/text/18/116 (accessed 16 November 2017).

9

Examination of the Nervous System

Graham M. Boswell

Department of Adult Nursing and Paramedic Science, Faculty of Education and Health, University of Greenwich, London, UK

9.1 General Examination

9.1.1 Introduction

The nervous system assessment constitutes an essential aspect in evaluating the patient's health. A neurological examination reveals the location and extent of lesions. Taking a history can also act as a guide in ordering and centralising the examination. Neural tissue comprises all components of the nervous system within the body. 'Neural tissue with supporting blood vessels and connective tissues form the organs of the nervous system including the brain, spinal cord, the receptors in complex sense organs such as the eye and ear and the nerves that link the nervous system with other systems' (Martini et al. 2012, p. 375). The nervous system in collaboration with the endocrine system share responsibility for maintaining homeostasis. (Tortora and Derrickson 2012). In addition to maintaining homeostasis, the nervous system is responsible for perception, behaviour and memory as well as initiating all voluntary

Pocket Guide to Physical Assessment, First Edition. Edited by Carol Lynn Cox.

Table 9.1 The brain.

Lobe	Functions the lobe is involved in
Frontal lobe	Motor function, mood, behaviour, decision making, memory, personality
Parietal lobe	Sensation, touch, pain, temperature, left/right determination
Temporal lobe	Hearing, language, memory, emotion, vision
Occipital lobe	Vision
Cerebellum	Modifies motor commands, balance, equilibrium, muscle tone

Table 9.2 Spinal nerves.

Region	Number
Cervical	8
Thoracic	12
Lumbar	5
Sacral	5
Coccygeal	1

movements (Tortora and Derrickson 2012). Changes in the nervous system affect other systems.

9.2 General Examination

Assessment of a patient's problem(s) is essential in planning effective care. An accurate history facilitates assessment of the pathology and helps guide the examination and identify appropriate tests. The examination reveals the location and extent of the lesion. The examination should address three questions: (i) Does the patient have a neurological illness? (ii) Where in the nervous system is the pathology located? (iii) What is the pathology? (Crossman and Neary 2014; Jarvis 2015; Swartz 2014).

The mnemonic SOCRATES is widely used to help explore symptoms especially pain (Table 9.3).

Table 9.3 SOCRATES.

S – Site	Where are the symptoms?
O – Onset	When did the symptoms begin?
C – Characteristics	If there is pain, is it dull, sharp, stabbing, burning, etc.?
R – Radiation	Is it localised, or does it spread and if so in what direction?
A – Associated factors	Any signs or symptoms associated with the pain?
T – Timing	Since it began, has it progressed?
E – Exacerbating or alleviating factors	Things that make the symptoms better or worse?
S – Severity	Grading symptoms such as pain scales, breathlessness, etc.

The following features in the history can be informative:

- speed of onset
  - rapid, abrupt – *vascular, oedema*, or *infective*
  - seconds – *seizure*
  - minutes – *migraine*
  - hours – *infective, inflammatory*
  - slow, progressive – *neoplasm* or *degenerative disorder*
- duration
  - brief episodes with recovery, e.g. *transient ischaemic attack (TIA), epilepsy, migraine, syncope*
  - longer episodes with recovery – *mechanical, obstruction*, or *pressure*
  - demyelination, e.g. *multiple sclerosis*
- frequency
- witness description – particularly if the patient has episodic loss of consciousness or is confused (Ball et al. 2014; Bickley and Szilagyi 2013; Japp and Robertson 2013; Jarvis 2015; Sirven and Malamut 2008; Swartz 2014; Talley and O'Connor 2013).

The minute examination of the nervous system can be elaborated almost indefinitely. Of far greater importance is to acquire the ability to conduct a thorough but comparatively rapid examination with confidence in the findings. As with other examinations, it is best to develop your own basic system and perform it consistently because this will help avoid omissions.

- Adapt your examination to the situation. The order in which functions are examined may be varied according to the symptoms, but the routine examination must be mastered.
  From the history, usually it will be obvious whether it is necessary to examine the mental functions in detail. A patient with sciatica would rightly be dismayed by an examination that began by asking him to name the parts of a watch.

The examination of the nervous system is approached under the following headings:

- Motor and sensory function
- Mental function
    - appearance and behaviour
    - mood
    - orientation
    - geographical orientation
    - memory
    - intelligence
    - speech and comprehension
- Cranial nerves (Ball et al. 2014; Bickley and Szilagyi 2013; Japp and Robertson 2013; Jarvis 2015; Sirven and Malmut 2008; Swartz 2014; Talley and O'Connor 2013).

9.3 Motor and Sensory Function

The motor examination should be carried out in a systematic way. You should begin by assessing the upper limbs to the neck and trunk and finally to the lower extremities of the patient. When examining the limbs and the trunk you will need to observe the patient's posture, muscle tone, presence or absence of involuntary movements, and muscular wasting and/or fasciculation. Your limb evaluation and examination should proceed from proximal to distal. Assess the major muscle groups first and if you note problems in any particular area then carry out a more detailed examination.

The assessment will examine the patient's proprioception, balance, gait, sensory stimuli, cortical sensory function, and reflex activity.

The nervous system cannot effectively be examined in isolation.

Other points of relevance may include:

- configuration of the skull and spine
- neck stiffness
- ear drums for otitis media
- blood pressure
- heart, e.g. arrhythmia, mitral stenosis
- carotid arteries – palpation and bruit
- neoplasms – breast, lung, abdominal
- jaundice.

9.4 Mental Function

9.4.1 General Observation

- appearance, e.g. unkempt
- behaviour, e.g. bewildered, restless, agitated
- emotional state, e.g. depressed, euphoric, hostile.

Observe, and ask for comments from nurses, other healthcare practitioners, and relatives.

9.4.2 Consciousness Level

If the patient is not fully conscious shake him gently and/or speak to him loudly but clearly. Record:

- drowsy but able to rouse to normal level
- drowsy but not able to rouse.

9.4.3 Glasgow Coma Scale (Appendix F)

The Glasgow coma scale (GCS) provides a rapid, widely used assessment of a patient's level of consciousness (Table 9.4). The GCS is an indirect measure of consciousness because it measures behaviours that are associated with conscious activity. Patterns of change in these behaviours when linked with alterations with pupil size, temperature, pulse, respirations, and blood pressure provide an effective guide to the extent of damage within the central nervous system. These observations can be even more effective when computer tomography (CT) and magnetic resonance imaging (MRI) scan evidence is also utilised.

Monitor responses to verbal command and if there is no response then a painful stimulus should be utilised. The painful stimuli should elicit a localising response which requires a central application. The trapezius pinch is the preferred option and is produced by squeezing the trapezius muscle between the thumb and index finger. Supraorbital pressure is usually the secondary choice for painful stimuli. Locate the supraorbital notch by feeling along the supraorbital arch at the nasal end and apply pressure with the thumb. If there is a risk of facial fractures this is contraindicated. The sternal rub (with knuckles over sternum) will damage the patient's skin and should be used only

Table 9.4 Glasgow Coma Scale (GCS).

Scoring the GCS	
There are three subscales: Eye opening (4), Verbal response (5), and Motor response (6). Each subscale must score a minimum of 1 to a maximum of 4–6 depending upon the subscale. This provides a score range of 3–15. A score between 3 and 8 necessitates airway management and a rapidly deteriorating score such as 2 points between observations requires urgent intervention.	
A Eye opening	4 – Spontaneous with normal blinking
	3 – Eyes open to command
	2 – Eyes open to pain
	1 – Eyes remain closed
B Verbal response	5 – Normal speech – able to hold a reasonable and relevant conversation
	4 – Confused speech – language is in a reasonable structure for the conversation but the meaning is inappropriate
	3 – Inappropriate words – single words spoken (expressing cerebral irritation) but no conversational structure
	2 – Incomprehensible sounds – moaning sounds only
	1 – No response
C Motor response	6 – Voluntary – responds normally to commands
	5 – Localising – attempts to protect site of pain
	4 – Flexion response – normal withdrawal of limb to pain
	3 – Abnormal flexion – exaggerated withdrawal of limb to pain with shoulder and elbow moving to the midline
	2 – Extension response to pain – adduction and internal rotation at shoulder, extension at elbows, pronation of forearms
	1 – No response

in extremis. Nail bed pressure (with smooth round object such as a torch) is sometimes used if there is no localising response to indicate that the limb is able to move but because this may be due to a spinal arc reflex it is an unreliable measure of cerebral function.

The GCS is the total score for the patient's response, but when communicating the GCS also provide the breakdown of scores as this ensures greater clarity for other healthcare professionals.

9.4.4 Confusion

If a patient appears confused, move on to assess cognitive state, including disorientation.

9.4.5 Language/Speech

Assess from conversation:

- Is there difficulty in articulation?
  If necessary, ask patient to say for example 'British Constitution', 'West Register Street'.
  - Dysarthria – difficulty moving and controlling the muscles of the lips, face, tongue, and the upper respiratory system that control speech.
  - Cerebellar or ataxic dysarthria – The cerebellum processes proprioceptive information that refines muscle activity in speech. Damage may result in scanning (slow, deliberate speech with each syllable equally stressed) or the voice may have a drunken quality, i.e. slurred because of the distorted vowels.
  - Lower motor neuron or flaccid dysarthria – Either bulbar or peripheral nerve lesions affect the muscles of articulation which may result in a rasping or monotonous voice, tongue wasting, and reduced lip control.

  - Upper motor neuron or spastic dysarthria – Damage to the pyramidal and extrapyramidal tracts affects muscle tone and strength especially of the lips and tongue. This results in slow speech, which requires more effort to produce and has a 'harsh' vocal quality.
- Is there altered voice tone?
  - extrapyramidal (monotonous and slow)
  - lower motor neuron (slurred)
  - upper motor neuron (slurred)
  - acute alcohol poisoning (slurred)
  - dysphonia – disorder of voice
    - cord lesion – hoarse
    - hysterical dysphonia is a stress related difficulty
- Is there difficulty in finding the right word?
  - dysphasia or aphasia – disorder of the use of words as symbols in speech, writing, and understanding; nearly always the result of left hemisphere lesion
    N.B. The centres for language are in people's dominant hemisphere. In right-handed and 75% of left-handed people, the dominant hemisphere is the left.
    - expressive dysphasia or slight dysphasia – difficult to detect; look for mispronounced words and circumlocutions in spontaneous speech; test for nominal aphasia by asking patient to name objects you point to, e.g. wristwatch, pen, chair, etc.; understanding should be intact
    - receptive dysphasia – speech fluent, but comprehension poor; patient may seem 'confused'; test for by asking patient to follow commands – a three-step

command is a good screening test (e.g. 'please pick up the glass, but first point to the curtain and then the door'); caused by a lesion in Wernicke's area
    - gross dysphasia or missed dysphasia – most common; usually obvious; the patient's spontaneous speech will be scanty, small vocabulary, often with the wrong words used; there are also other dysphasias produced by interruption of the connecting pathways between the speech centres
- aphasia or mutism – no speech at all, just grunts; this may be due to aphasia, anarthria, psychiatric disease, or occasionally diffuse cerebral pathology (Ball et al. 2014; Bickley and Szilagyi 2013; Japp and Robertson 2013; Jarvis 2015; Sirven et al. 2008; Swartz 2014; Talley and O'Connor 2013).

9.4.6 Other Defects Occurring in Absence Motor or Sensory Dysfunction

9.4.6.1 First Establish the Normal Reading and Writing Skills of the Person

- dyslexia – inappropriate difficulty with reading; read few lines from newspaper (having established that comprehension and expressive speech are intact)
- dysgraphia – inappropriate difficulty writing
- agraphia – loss of ability to write
- acalculia – loss of ability to do mental and written sums
- apraxia – inability to perform a learned purposeful task when there is no paralysis, e.g. opening matchbox, waving goodbye; apraxia for dressing is common in *diffuse brain disease*

- visual agnosia – inability to visually recognise familiar objects
- auditory agnosia – inability to recognise familiar sounds
- astereognosis – tactile agnosia – With their eyes closed, it is the inability to recognise common objects (e.g. a key or coin when placed in the hand)
- parietal lobe lesions – can cause a neglect of the opposite side of the body, there are no perceived sensations and so the half of the body is not recognised by the conscious brain; right parietal lobe lesions cause particular problems with spatial awareness: getting lost in familiar places, inability to lay table, to draw or make patterns, and neglect of left side of space (Ball et al. 2014; Bickley and Szilagyi 2013; Japp and Robertson 2013; Jarvis 2015; Sirven et al. 2008; Swartz 2014; Talley and O'Connor 2013).

9.4.7 Cognitive Function

Take account of any evidence you have about the patient's intelligence, education, and interests.

'Cognitive' is a term that covers orientation, thought processes, and logic.

9.4.7.1 Orientation

In the process of normal conversation, you can check the patient's awareness of time, place, and person. The ability to respond and contribute appropriately to a conversation with the consequent changes of parameters inherent to a 'normal' conversation would indicate that understanding (Wernicke's area) and speech (Broca's area) are able to function. Issues of time, place, and person provide some details that you may find easier to check but which require less use of the patient's language centres. The patient's sentence construction demonstrates how well the speech process is working; therefore, questions that require one-word answers should be avoided.

Disorientation indicates disruption of the pathways between language understanding and expression. *Depressed patients* may be unwilling to reply although they know the answers.

9.4.7.2 Attention and Calculation

- Test the concentration of a patient by asking them to take away 7 from 100, 7 from 93, etc. or by asking them to say the months of the year backwards.

Concentration may be impaired with many cerebral abnormalities, depression, and anxiety.

9.4.7.3 Memory (Appendix E: Mini-Mental State Examination)

9.4.7.3.1 Immediate Recall – Digit Span

- Ask the patient to repeat a random series of numbers. Speak slowly and start with an easy short sequence and then increase the numbers. Most people manage seven digits' forwards, five backwards.

9.4.7.3.2 Short-Term Memory

- Ask patient to tell you:
    - what they had for breakfast
    - what they did the night before
    - what they read in today's paper.

      Demented patients will be unable to do this. They may confabulate (make up impressive stories) to cover their difficulty.

9.4.7.3.3 New Memory

- Ask patient in early part of your assessment to remember four or five common objects such as orange, apple, pen, book, and teddy bear, make sure the patient has learnt it. After 10 minutes or so ask the patient to recall your objects. It is a good idea to note the objects and order.

9.4.7.3.4 Longer-Term Memory

- Ask patient and if necessary check with relatives, etc.
    - events before illness, e.g. last year, or during last week
    - 'What is your address?'

9.4.7.3.5 General Knowledge

- Assess in relation to anticipated performance from history.
    - What is the name of the President/Prime Minister or other political leader.
    - Name six capital cities.
    - What were the dates of a major event relevant to the patient's societal grouping that happened approximately two to five years ago. You may need to ask about several events because depending upon the questions, a person's inability to answer may just reflect a lack of interest rather than an inability to recall.
    - In *acute organic states* and *dementia*, new learning, recent memory, and reasoning are usually more impaired than remote memory. Vocabulary is usually well preserved in *dementia*. In *depression*, patients may be unwilling to reply, and appear demented.
    - A history from a relative or employer is very important in early dementia (Ball et al. 2014; Bickley and Szilagyi 2013; Japp and Robertson 2013; Jarvis 2015; Sirven et al. 2008; Swartz 2014; Talley and O'Connor 2013).

9.4.7.3.6 Reasoning (Abstract Thought)

- What does this proverb mean: 'Let sleeping dogs lie?'. An adult is normally able to give an abstract explanation of the proverb. If they give a concrete explanation it may indicate impaired cerebral function such as early dementia.

9.5 Skull and Spine

- Inspect and palpate skull if there is any possibility of a head injury.
- Check neck stiffness – meningeal irritation.
- Inspect spine – usually when examining back of chest.
- If there is any possibility of pathology, stand patient and check all movements of spine; if there is possible trauma then X-ray first.

9.6 Cranial Nerves (I–XII)

- Examine cranial nerves and upper limbs with patient sitting up, preferably on side of bed or on a chair (Table 9.5).

9.6.1 I Olfactory Nerve

Not normally tested unless there are other neurological deficits, including papilloedema, undiagnosed headache (especially frontal), or head injury. Ask the patient to close eyes, then close one nostril by palpation. Then present a smell such as oil of cloves, peppermint, coffee, etc. to the open nostril. Test each nostril in turn. It is normal not to be able to name all smells, but one smell should be distinguished from another. Pungent or noxious smells such as ammonia should not be used, as they are perceived by the fifth cranial nerve and confuse results. A loss of the sensation of smell (anosmia) indicates possible:

- *base of skull fracture*	especially if loss of smell is one sided
- *olfactory groove meningioma*	especially if loss of smell is one sided
- *rhinitis*	more likely if loss of smell is bilateral
- *smoking*	more likely if loss of smell is bilateral

Table 9.5 'Examine the cranial nerves'.

I	Olfactory	Smell
II	Optic	Visual acuity
		Visual field
		Fundi
III, IV, and VI	Occulomotor, trochlear, and abducens	Ptosis
		Nystagmus
		Eye movements
		Pupils
V	Trigeminal	Facial sensation
		Corneal reflex
		Jaw muscles/jerk
		Tongue taste
VII	Facial	Face muscles
VIII	Vestibuloauditory	Hearing
		Rinne/Weber tests
		Nystagmus/gait
IX, X	Glossopharyngeal, vagus	Palate
		Swallowing
		Taste – posterior third of tongue
XI	Spinal accessory	Trapezius
XII	Hypoglossal	Tongue wasting

9.6.2 II Optic Nerve

9.6.2.1 Visual Acuity (Appendixes A and B Acuity Charts)

- Test each eye separately.
- Check patient can read a language you understand and then ask them to read small text such

as newspaper print with each eye separately, with reading glasses if used.

- If sight poor, test formally:
  - near vision – newsprint or Jaeger type (each eye in turn) (see Appendix A)
  - distant vision – Snellen type (more precise method) (see Appendix B)
    Stand patient at 6 m from Snellen's card (each eye in turn). Results expressed as a ratio:
    - 6 – distance of person from card
    - x – distance at which patient should be able to read type
      i.e. 6/6 is good vision, 6/60 means the smallest type the patient can read is large enough to be normally read at 60 m.
      If the patient cannot read 6/6, try after correction with glasses or pinhole. Looking through a pinhole in a card obviates refractive errors, analogous to a pinhole camera. If vision remains poor, suspect a neurological or ophthalmic cause.
      A 3 m Snellen chart is shown in Appendix B.
      A pinhole is not effective for correcting near vision for reading.

9.6.2.2 Visual Fields

- Quick method for temporal peripheral patient fields by confrontation of patient and examiner with both eyes open. Always test fields. Patients are often unaware of visual loss, the most dramatic of which is Anton's syndrome (blindness with lack of awareness of the blindness).
  - Sit opposite the patient and ask them to look at your nose with both eyes open.

- Examine each eye in turn.
- Bring waggling finger forwards from behind patient's ear in upper and lower lateral quadrants and ask when it can be seen.
    - Normal vision is approximately 100° from axis of eye.
      The patient must fully understand the test. The extreme of peripheral vision can be tested with both eyes open, because the nose obstructs vision from the other eye. If peripheral field seems restricted, retest with the other eye covered to ensure each eye is being tested separately.
- A peripheral defect in the visual field of one eye would indicate a nasal defect in the other eye. To test this, the patient covers the eye with the peripheral defect and then the examiner moves the waggling finger from the expected defect towards the area of better vision.
- Normal vision is approximately 50° from each axis of eye.

- Standard method for examination:
  Hold a small red pinhead in the plane midway between the patient and examiner. With the other eye covered, compare the visual fields of the patient with that of the examiner, with a pin brought in from temporal or nasal fields.
- Defects in the central field can be assessed by the standard method with a small red pin held in the plane midway between the patient and examiner:
    - scotoma – defects in the central field (*retinal or optic nerve lesion*)
    - enlarged blind spot (*papilloedema*)

  Map by moving the pin from inside scotoma or blind spot outwards until red pinhead reappears.

  This is a crude test and small areas of loss of vision may need to be formally tested with a perimetry test.

- Test for sensory inattention when fields are full with both eyes open.
  - Hold your hands between you and the patient, one opposite each ear and waggle forefingers simultaneously. Ask which moves. With a parietal defect, the patient may not recognise movement on one side, although fields are full to formal testing.

    The patterns of visual field deficit will indicate where the lesion is on the optic pathway from the optic disc to the occipital cortex. The changes in the visual field deficit occur because at the optic chiasma half of the optic nerve crosses over to enable stereoptic vision. A review of visual pathways is that all light from the right reaches the left-hand side of both optic discs and then travels to the left occipital cortex (blue) and vice versa. Deficits before the optic chiasma (1) cause problems in one eye only. Deficits at the optic chiasma are usually central (2 – bitemporal hemianopia) and caused by an enlarged pituitary (such as pituitary adenoma). At the optic chiasma the problems are mirrored in both visual fields whereas after the optic chiasma the deficits affect one side of the visual field in both eyes (3, 4, and 5). Partial damage to the optic radiation will produce a partial deficit (4), with a top-quadrant defect being caused by temporal damage or an occipital lesion and a lower-quadrant defect being caused by parietal damage or an occipital lesion (Figure 9.1).

9.6.2.3 Examine the Fundi

- Lesions particularly relevant to the neurological system:
  - *optic atrophy* – pale disc and demyelination, e.g. *multiple sclerosis: pressure on nerve*

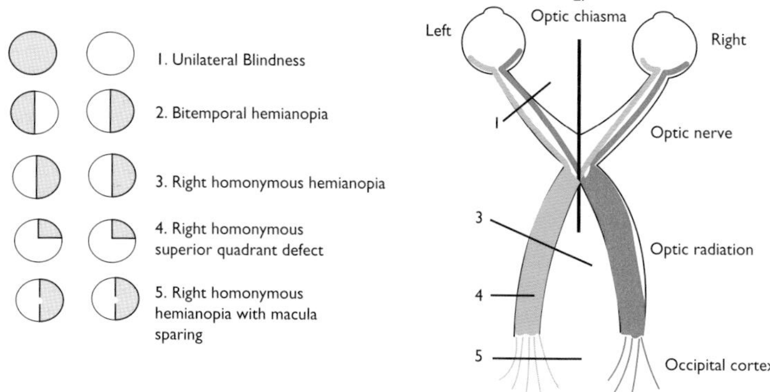

Figure 9.1 Visual Field Defects. Source: Boswell 2004.

- *papilloedema* – caused by a raised intracranial pressure (RICP); RICP pushes cerebral tissue through the superior orbital fissure, which squashes the back of the eye; this is more likely with conditions that cause acute changes in intracranial pressure such as *tumours, trauma*, and *obstructive hydrocephalus*

- Nystagmus – a sensitive test for nystagmus is to ask the patient to cover the other eye during fundoscopy. This removes fixation and can help to elicit nystagmus.

9.6.3 II Optic Nerve and III Oculomotor Nerve

Assessment of the cranial nerves related to the eye and eye function will have a degree of overlap: a constriction of a pupil to light involves the optic nerve transmitting the light stimuli and the oculomotor nerve stimulating the pupils to constrict.

- Look at pupils. Are they round and equal? (Normal pupils for adults are between 2 and 5 mm in diameter.)

- Symmetric small pupils: (< 2 mm)
    - *old age*
    - *opiates*
    - *Argyll Robertson pupils (syphilis)* are small, irregular, eccentric pupils, reacting to convergence but not light
    - pilocarpine eye drops for *narrow-angle glaucoma*
- Symmetric large pupils: (> 6 mm)
    - *youth*
    - *alcohol*
    - *sympathomimetics, anxiety*
    - *atropine-like substances*
- Asymmetric pupils (anisocoria):
    - *3rd-nerve palsy* – affected pupil dilated, often with ptosis and diplopia
    - *Horner's syndrome* (sympathetic defect) – affected pupil constricted (miosis – smaller pupil), often with partial ptosis (drooping eye lid), enophthalmos (backward displacement of the eyeball into the orbit) and anhydrosis (abnormal deficiency of sweat)
    - *iris trauma*
    - *drugs* (see above) – e.g. tropicamide 1.0% or cyclopentolate 1.0% will be used in the treatment of anterior uveitis

- Light reflex: Shine bright light from torch into each pupil in turn in a dimly lit room. Do pupils contract equally?
    - *Holmes–Adie pupil*: large, slowly reacting to light
    - *afferent defect, ocular or optic nerve blindness*: neither pupil responds to light in blind eye; both conditions respond to light in normal eye (consensual response in blind eye)
    - relative afferent defect – direct response appears normal but when light moves from normal to deficient eye, paradoxical dilation of pupil occurs

    - *efferent defect–3rd-nerve lesion*, pupil does not respond to light in either eye
- Accommodation reflex: Ask patient to look at distant object, and then at your finger 10–15 cm from nose – do pupils contract?
    - Response to accommodation but not light:
        - *Argyll Robertson*
        - *Holmes–Adie*
        - *occular blindness*
        - *midbrain lesion*
        - some recovering *3rd-nerve lesions*

9.6.4 III Oculomotor Nerve, IV Trochlear Nerve and VI Abducens Nerve

Smooth movement of the eye is achieved through the opposing muscles equally contracting and relaxing, a process controlled by three cranial nerves. The oculomotor (III) controls the superior, medial, and inferior rectus; the inferior oblique; pupil; and the levator palpebrae (raises upper eyelid). Moving the eye up, down, and inwards to the nose. The trochlear (IV) controls the superior oblique and moves the eye up and out. The abducens (VI) controls the lateral rectus and moves the eye out.

9.6.4.1 External Ocular Movements

- Test the eye movements in the four cardinal directions (left, right, up, and down as though you were printing a large H in the air) and convergence using your finger at 1 m distance.

Look for abnormal eye movements. Testing external ocular movements (EOM).

- Ask: ‘Tell me if you see double’.
  Upward gaze and convergence are often reduced in uncooperative patients.

- To detect minor lesions:
  - Find direction of gaze with maximum separation of images.
  - Cover one eye and ask which image has gone. Peripheral image is seen by the eye that is not moving fully.

    Peripheral image is displaced in direction of action of weak muscle, e.g. maximum diplopia on gaze to left. Left eye sees peripheral image, which is displaced laterally. Therefore, left lateral rectus is weak.
- Diplopia may be due to a single muscle or nerve lesion (N.B. monocular diplopia usually implies ocular pathology):
  - paralytic strabismus (squint)
    - III palsy: diploplia, ptosis (drooping eye lid), large fixed pupil, eye can be abducted only; eye is often looking 'down and outwards'
    - IV palsy: diplopia when eye looks down or inwards
    - VI palsy: abduction paralysed, diplopia when looking to side of lesion
  - concomitant nonparalytic strabismus, e.g. *childhood ocular lesion* – constant angle between eyes. Usually no double vision as one eye ignored (amblyopic).
  - conjugate ocular palsy
    - *supranuclear palsies* affecting coordination rather than muscle weakness; inability to look in particular direction, usually upwards
    - *intranuclear lesion*: convergence normal but cannot adduct eyes on lateral gaze
  - if patient sees double in all directions
    - may be *3rd-nerve palsy*
    - *thyroid muscle disease* – worse in morning

- *myasthenia gravis* – worse in evening
- manifest strabismus.

9.6.4.2 Ptosis

Drooping of upper eyelid can be:

- complete – *third-nerve palsy*
- incomplete
  - *partial third-nerve palsy*
  - muscular weakness, e.g. *myasthenia gravis* (from anti-acetylcholine receptor antibodies)
  - sympathetic tone decreased – *Horner's syndrome* (also small pupils – miosis and enophthalmos and decreased sweating on face)
  - partial Horner's syndrome (small irregular pupils with ptosis) in *autonomic neuropathy* of *diabetes* and *syphilis*
  - lid swelling
  - *levator dysinsertion syndrome* (from chronic contact lens use)

9.6.4.3 Nystagmus

This is an involuntary rapid back and forth movement of the eye in a horizontal, vertical, or a combination of directions. Nystagmus is labelled by the direction of the fast movement (the return movement is a little slower). A small amount of end-position (at the extremes of gaze) lateral nystagmus is normal. Horizontal nystagmus is often associated with problems in the labyrinth and vertical nystagmus frequently with brain stem problems. (Swartz 2014)

- Test first in the neutral position and then with the eyes deviated to right, left, and upwards. Keep object within binocular field as nystagmus is often normal in extremes of gaze. Keep your movements smooth.
  - cerebellar nystagmus.

  - fast movement to side of gaze (on both sides)
  - increased when looking to lesion
  - *cerebellar* or *brainstem lesion* or *drugs* (*ethanol, phenytoin*)
- vestibular nystagmus
  - fast movement only in one direction – away from lesion
  - reduced by fixation if peripheral in origin
  - more marked when looking away from lesion
  - *inner ear, vestibular disease* or *brain-stem lesion*

    Labyrinthine nystagmus may be positional – particularly in benign positional vertigo and can be induced by hyperextension and rotation of the neck (Hallpike manoeuvre) which after a latency of a few seconds will produce a vertical/torsional type of nystagmus for about 10–15 seconds, along with symptoms of vertigo.
- congenital nystagmus – constant horizontal wobbling
- downbeat nystagmus – foramen magnum lesion or Wernicke's disease
- retraction nystagmus – midbrain lesion
- complex nystagmus – brainstem disease, usually multiple sclerosis

9.6.4.4 Saccades

This is the rapid eye movement used to change eye position. It is tested in the horizontal and vertical planes by asking the patient to switch fixation between two targets (e.g. the examiner's fingers). Slow saccades may be seen in a variety of disorders including degenerative disorders such as progressive supranuclear palsy.

9.6.5 V Trigeminal Nerve

9.6.5.1 *Sensory V*

- Test light touch in all three divisions with cotton wool. Ask the patient to close his eyes and to tell you when and where he is being touched. Pinprick usually only if needed to delineate anaesthetic area.

Corneal Reflex–Sensory V (Trigeminal) and Motor VII (Facial)

- Ask the patient to look up and away from you and touch the cornea from the opposite side to the gaze, with a wisp of cotton wool. Both eyes should blink. The corneal reflex is easily prompted incorrectly by eliciting the 'eyelash' or 'menace' reflex.

9.6.5.2 *Motor V – Muscles of Jaw*

- Ask the patient to open their mouth against resistance and look to see if the jaw descends in midline. Palsy of the nerve causes deviation of the jaw to the side of the lesion. Fifth-nerve palsies are very rare in isolation.
- Jaw jerk – only if other neurological findings, e.g. upper motor neuron lesion. Increased jaw jerk is only present if there is a bilateral upper motor neuron fifth-nerve lesion, e.g. *bilateral strokes* or *pseudobulbar palsy.*
    - Put your forefinger gently on the patient's loosely opened jaw. Tap your finger gently with a tendon hammer. Explain the test to the patient or relaxation of the jaw will be impossible. A brisk jerk is a positive finding.

9.6.6 VII Facial Nerve

- Ask the patient to:
  - raise eyebrows
  - close eyes tightly
  - smile
  - frown
  - show you their teeth
  - puff out cheeks

  Demonstrate these to the patient yourself if necessary.

  Lower motor neuron lesion: all muscles on the side of the lesion are affected, e.g. *Bell's palsy*: widened palpebral fissure, weak blink, drooped mouth.

  Upper motor neuron lesion: only the lower muscles are affected, i.e. mouth drops to one side but eyebrows raise normally. This is because the upper half of the face is bilaterally innervated. This abnormality is very common in a hemiparesis.
- Taste – can be tested easily only on anterior two-thirds of tongue.
  Ask patient to close eyes and stick their tongue out, small amounts of glucose (sweet), lemon (sour) or sodium chloride (salt) in solution can be placed on the tongue.

9.6.7 VIII Vestibuloauditory Nerve

9.6.7.1 Vestibular

No easy bedside test for this nerve except looking for nystagmus.

9.6.7.2 Acoustic

- Block one ear by pressing the tragus. Whisper numbers increasingly loudly in the other ear until the patient can repeat them.

More accurate tests are as follows:

- Rinne's test. Compares a patient's hearing of a tone conducted via the bone and air. Place a high-pitched vibrating tuning fork on the mastoid. When the patient says the sound stops, hold the fork 1 in. from the external auditory meatus. Ask the patient whether the tone is louder at point 1(bone) or point 2 (air).
    - If there is nerve deafness then the tone is audible at the external auditory meatus because air and bone conduction will be reduced equally. As such air conduction will be better than bone conduction (as it would be normally). A positive Rinne's test.
    - If the tone is not heard at the external auditory meatus then bone conduction is better than air conduction (conductive hearing loss). A negative Rinne's test
- Weber's test. Hold a lightly vibrating tuning fork firmly on the top of the patient's head or on the forehead. The sound should be heard equally in both ears. If the sound is heard to one side, either there is a conductive hearing loss on that side or there is a sensorineural hearing loss on the other side.

9.6.8 IX Glossopharyngeal

- Ask patient to say 'Ahh' and watch for symmetrical upwards movement of uvula – pulled away from weak side.
- Touch the back of the pharynx with an orange stick or spatula gently. If the patient gags the nerve is intact.

  This gag reflex depends on the IX and X nerve, the former being the sensory side and the latter the motor aspect. It is frequently absent with ageing and abuse of tobacco.

9.6.9 X Vagus Nerve

- Ask if the patient can swallow normally.
  There are so many branches of the vagus nerve that it is impossible to be sure it is all functioning normally. If the vagus nerve is seriously damaged, swallowing is a problem; spillage into the lungs may occur. Swallowing can be assessed by initially ensuring that cranial nerves V, VII, IX, and XII are working correctly (oral stage) and listening and watching a person talk will give a good indication of the function of these cranial nerves. Then asking the patient to swallow (without food or fluid), the pharyngeal stage lasts one second. Observe that the throat muscles (pharyngeal constrictor muscles) move evenly, effectively, and at normal speed. If the dry swallow is effective, then ask the patient to take a small drink of water. Coughing on attempted swallow indicates a high risk of aspiration. Check speech afterwards. A change of voice quality ('wet' speech) indicates pooling of fluids on the vocal cords and indicates a high risk of aspiration. Check for a voluntary cough as this can become quiet and ineffective. Check speech for dysarthria. Whenever patients have been intubated and had an endotracheal tube in situ, a swallowing assessment should be undertaken before fluids or food is given by mouth to ensure aspiration is prevented.

9.6.10 XI Spinal Accessory Nerve

- Ask the patient to flex neck, pressing the chin against your resisting hand. Observe if both sternomastoids contract normally.
- Ask the patient to raise both shoulders. If they cannot, the trapezius muscle is not functioning.

Failure of the trapezius muscle on one side is often associated with a *hemiplegia* (particularly anterior cerebral artery infarctions).

- Ask the patient to turn their head against your resisting hand. This tests the contralateral sternomastoid and can help to demonstrate normal motor functioning in a *hysterical hemiplegia*.

9.6.11 XII Hypoglossal Nerve

- Ask the patient to put out their tongue. If it protrudes to one side, this is the side of the weakness, e.g. deviating to left on protrusion from left hypoglossal lesion.
- Look for fasciculation or wasting with mouth open.

9.7 Limbs and Trunk

9.7.1 General Inspection

- Look at the patient's resting and standing posture:
    - flexed upper limb, extended lower limb – *hemiplegia*
    - wrist drop – *radial nerve palsy*
- Look for abnormal movements:
    - tremor
        - *Parkinson's* – coarse rhythmical tremor at rest, lessens on movement
        - *essential tremor* (*thyrotoxicosis*) – tremor present on action; look at outstretched hands
    - *chorea* – abrupt, involuntary repetitive semi-purposeful movement
    - *athetosis* – slow, continuous writhing movement of limb
    - *spasm* – exaggerated, involuntary muscular contraction

- Look for muscle wasting. Check distribution:
    - symmetrical, e.g. *Duchenne muscular dystrophy*
    - asymmetrical, e.g. *poliomyelitis*
    - proximal, e.g. *limb-girdle muscular dystrophy*
    - distal, e.g. *peripheral neuropathy*
    - generalised, e.g. *motor neuron disease*
    - localised, e.g. with *joint disease*
- Look for fasciculation. This is irregular involuntary contractions of small bundles of muscle fibres, not perceived by the patient.
  This is typical of denervation, e.g. *motor neuron disease* when it is widespread. It is caused by the death of anterior horn cells.

9.7.2 Arms

9.7.2.1 Inspection

In addition to the general inspection it is important to make an initial assessment.

- Ask the patient to hold both arms straight out in front them with palms up and eyes shut. Observe gross weakness and posture and whether the arms remain stationary:
    - hypotonic posture – wrist flexed and fingers extended
    - drift – gradually upwards with sensory loss, may be *cerebellar damage*
    - gradually downwards may be *pyramidal weakness*
    - downwards without pronation can be seen in *hysteria* or in profound *proximal muscle weakness*
    - athetoid tremors – *sensory loss* (peripheral nerve) or *cerebellar disease*
- Tap both arms downwards. They should by reflex return to their former position.

If the arm overswings in its return to its position, weakness or *cerebellar dysfunction* may be present.

- Ask the patient to do fast finger movements. Quickly touch each fingertip on one hand to the thumb and repeat several times, or ask them to pretend they are playing a fast tune on the piano. You may have to demonstrate this yourself. Clumsy movements can be a sensitive index of a slight *pyramidal lesion*. The dominant side should always be quicker than the nondominant side.

9.7.2.2 Coordination

- Ask the patient to touch their nose with index finger.
- With the patient's eyes open, ask them to touch their nose, then your finger, which is held up in front of the patient. This can be repeated rapidly with your finger moving from place to place in front of the patient, but your finger must be in position before the patient's finger leaves their nose.

  Past pointing (missing your finger) and marked intention tremor in the absence of muscular weakness suggests *cerebellar dysfunction*. If you suspect a cerebellar abnormality check rapid alternating movements (*dysdiadochokinesia*):

  - fast rotation of the hands on the patient's lap (supination and pronation)
  - tapping back of other hand as quickly as possible

    Damage to the cerebellum results in a loss of proprioception, the brain's unconsciousness awareness of the position of the joints, muscles, and limbs. Proprioception enables normal movement to be a smoothly coordinated process. Any disruption creates clumsiness, especially at night when vision is less able to compensate (Swartz 2014).

9.7.2.3 *Tone*

(Refer to the Musculoskeletal Examination for examples of assessment.)

Always check tone before you assess strength. This is a difficult test to perform as patients often do not relax. Try to distract the patient with conversation.

- Ask the patient to relax the arm and then you flex and extend the wrist or elbow. Move through a wide arc moderately slowly, at irregular intervals to prevent patient cooperation.
- Ask the patient to let the leg go loose, lift it up, and move at the knee joint (hip and ankle if required). It can be difficult to assess this in the legs because patients often cannot relax. Ankle clonus can be assessed at the same time (refer to examination technique below).

  Hypertonia (increased tone):
  - pyramidal: more obvious in flexion of upper limbs and extension of lower limbs; occasionally 'clasp knife', i.e. diminution of tone during movement
  - extrapyramidal: uniform 'lead pipe' rigidity. If associated with tremor the movement feels like a 'cog wheel'
  - hysterical: increases with increased movement

  Hypotonia (decreased tone):

  lower motor neuron lesion
  recent upper motor neuron lesion
  cerebellar lesion
  unconsciousness

9.7.2.4 *Muscle Power*

For screening purposes, examine two distal muscles, one flexor and one extensor (e.g. finger flexion and extension), and two proximal muscles in each limb. Compare each side. Confirm the weakness suspected by palpation of the muscle.

Strength/power is usually graded:

0. No active contraction.
1. Visible as palpable contraction with *no* active movement.
2. Movement with gravity eliminated, i.e. in horizontal direction.
3. Movement against gravity.
4. Movement against gravity plus resistance.
5. Normal power.

- Look for patterns of weakness:
  - *hemiplegia* – muscles weak all down one side
  - *monoplegia* – weakness of one limb
  - *paraplegia* – weakness of both lower limbs
  - *tetraplegia* – weakness of all four limbs
  - *myasthenia* – weakness developing after repeated contractions – most obvious in smaller muscles, e.g. repeated blinking
  - proximal muscles, e.g. *myopathy*
  - nerve root distribution, e.g. *disc prolapse*
  - nerve distribution, e.g. wrist drop from *radial nerve palsy*

9.7.2.5 Upper Limbs

- As indicated previously, compare each side and confirm the weakness suspected by palpation of the muscle. For example:
  - 'Squeeze my fingers'. Present the two forefingers of each hand. The patient may hurt you if they squeeze your whole hand.
  - Ask the patient to extend arms (demonstrate) and then say, 'Stop me pressing them down'.

  - Ask the patient to bend the arm and as you hold the wrist ask him to force the arm down against resistance to check extension.
- Resistance to extension:
  - Ask patient to bend the arm and as you hold the wrist ask them to pull the arm up against resistance to check flexion.

    Gross power loss will have been noted on inspection of extended arm position or on walking.
- If the patient is in bed, start the examination by asking them to:
  - raise both arms
  - raise one leg off the bed
- Test power at joints against your own strength – shoulder, elbow, wrist.
  - power at main joints cannot normally be overcome by permissible force.
- If there is weakness or other neurological signs in a limb, test the individual muscle groups:
  - shoulder – abduction, extension, flexion
  - elbow – flexion, extension
  - wrist – flexion, extension: 'Hold wrists up, do not let me push them down'.
  - finger – flexion, grasp, extension, adduction (put a piece of paper between straight fingers held in extension and ask the patient to hold it; *as you* remove it), abduction (with fingers in extension, ask patient to spread them apart against your force)

9.7.2.6 Tendon Reflexes

9.7.2.6.1 Arms

- Place arms comfortably by side with elbows flexed and hands on upper abdomen. Tell the patient to relax because reflexes are easier to see; continuing to talk with the patient during this part of the examination may provide distraction and help accuracy. Compare sides.

- supinator reflex: tap the distal end of the radius with a tendon hammer
- biceps reflex: tap your forefinger or thumb over biceps tendon
- triceps reflex: hold arm across chest to tap your thumb over the triceps tendon

Increased jerks – *upper motor neuron lesion* (e.g. hemiparesis).

Decreased jerks – *lower motor neuron lesion* or acute *upper motor neuron lesion.*

Clonus – pressure stretching a muscle group causes rhythmical involuntary contraction. If a brisk reflex is obtained, test for clonus. Found in *marked hypertonia* from stretching tendon. No need to strike tendon with tendon hammer. Clonus confirms an increased tendon jerk and suggests an upper motor neuron lesion. A few symmetrical beats may be normal.

9.7.2.6.2 Trunk

- The superficial abdominal reflexes rarely need to be tested.
  - Lightly stroke each quadrant with an orange stick or the back of your fingernail. Note the contractions of the muscles and movement of the umbilicus towards the stimulus. These reflexes are absent or decreased in an upper or lower motor neuron lesion.
- Cremasteric reflex T12–L1
  - Stroke inside of leg – induces testis to rise from cremaster muscle contraction.
- Palpate the bladder.
  The patient with a distended bladder will feel very uncomfortable as *you* palpate it.

Many neurological lesions, sensory or motor, will lead to a distended bladder, giving the patient *retention with overflow incontinence.*

- Examine the strength of the abdominal muscles by asking the patient to attempt to sit up without using hands.

9.8 Lower Limbs

9.8.1 Inspection

As for arms.

9.8.2 Coordination

- Ask the patient to run the heel of one leg up and down the shin of the other leg. Lack of coordination will be apparent.
  Gait may become broad based, and the patient may be unable to perform a tandem gait (heel–toe walking).

9.8.3 Tone

- Ask the patient to let limb go loose, lift it up, and move at knee joint (hip and ankle if required)
  It may be difficult to assess in the legs because patients may have difficulty relaxing. Ankle clonus can be assessed at the same time (see below).

9.8.4 Muscle Power

Bending and straightening the knee as well as dorsiflexion and plantarflexion of the ankle against resistance will demonstrate the muscle power in the legs. Lifting the straight leg off the bed against resistance will demonstrate hip flexion.

- hip flexion: ask the patient to lift leg, and say, 'Don't let me push it down'.
- hip extension: ask the patient to keep leg straight on the couch or bed surface and try to lift at the ankle; you can test for abduction and adduction against resistance as well; refer to Chapter 13 for further information on performing these tests.
- knee – flexion and extension
- ankle – plantarflexion, dorsiflexion, eversion, and inversion

Only severe weakness will be detected because the legs are stronger than the arms. If no weakness is detected and the patient is complaining of weakness, then more sensitive tests can be helpful, e.g. walking on tiptoes, heels, arising from a squat position, hopping on either leg.

Hip weakness is easily overlooked. If a weakness is suspected, test the patient's ability to lift their own weight, i.e. rising from a chair or climbing stairs.

Occasionally patients will have hysterical weakness. A useful test is Hoover's sign. This is tested by placing your hand under the ankle of the patient's paralysed leg. The patient is first asked to extend the paralysed leg (which should produce no effort), and then by asking for hip flexion of the nonparalysed leg, resulting in contraction of the 'paralysed' hip extensor (a reflex fixation that we all do). Unlike other tests for nonorganic illness, this test demonstrates normalcy in the paralysed limb (Jarvis 2015; Swartz 2014).

9.8.5 Tendon Reflexes

Deep tendon reflexes are tested to demonstrate how well the central nervous system is operating. In testing the patella reflex when the leg is relaxed and dangling the tendon is tapped – this suddenly stretches the tendon (as if the knee was further bent), the muscle spindles (stretch receptors) are stimulated and a spinal arc reflex is generated to effectively return the tendon (and therefore the lower leg) to the resting position but because the leg is still dangling the effect is to kick the lower leg forwards normally just a few inches. Reflexes are exaggerated in upper motor neuron damage because the spinal arc reflex operates without the cerebral controls. Reflexes are absent in lower motor neuron damage because the spinal arc reflex is interrupted.

Although muscle tone can increase in the older adult (reducing flexibility), the muscle power is mostly well preserved. Deep tendon reflexes do not normally diminish in the elderly, but ankle jerks may be compromised by inelasticity of the achilles tendon. As such, alteration of reflexes are indicative of disease (Sirven **and** Malamut 2008).

- Test knee reflexes by passing left forearm behind both knees, supporting them partly flexed. Ask the patient to let leg go loose and tap the tendons below patella.
    - Compare both sides.
      Reflexes can be normal, brisk (can occur in normal subjects or *upper motor* neuron lesion), decreased, absent (always abnormal).
- Test ankle reflex by flexing the knee and abducting the leg. Apply gentle pressure to the ball of the foot, with it at a right angle and tap the tendon.
  Ankle jerks are often absent in the elderly.
- Compare sides – right versus left and arms versus legs. It is essential that the patient is relaxed when reflexes are tested. This is not always easy for the patient, particularly the elderly. You can elicit reinforcement (an apparently absent reflex may become

present) by asking the patient to clasp his hands together and pull one hand against the other just as you strike with the hammer.

Increased jerks – *upper motor neuron lesion* (e.g. hemiparesis).

Decreased jerks – *lower motor neuron lesion* or *acute upper motor neuron lesion.*

Clonus – if a brisk reflex is obtained, test for clonus. A sharp, then sustained dorsiflexion of the foot by pressure on ball of the foot, may result in the foot 'beating' for many seconds. Clonus confirms an increased tendon jerk and suggests an *upper motor neuron lesion.* A few symmetrical beats may be normal.

9.8.6 Plantar Reflexes

- Tell patient what you are doing and scratch the side of the sole with a firm but not painful implement (orange stick or rounded spike on tendon hammer). Watch for flexion or extension of the toes.

  Normal plantar responses = flexion of all toes.

  Extensor (Babinski) response = slow extension of the big toe with spreading of the other toes. Withdrawal from pain or tickle is rapid and not abnormal. In individuals with sensitive feet, the reflex can be elicited by noxious stimuli elsewhere in the leg; stroking the lateral aspect of the foot can be very useful or testing for sharp sensation on the dorsum of the great toe. (Do not use needles or pins to test for 'pinprick' sensation. Use a disposable 'neurostick', 'neuropin', or paper clip and ask the patient to tell you whether the sensation is sharp or dull.)

  An extensor reflex is normal up to six months of age.

9.8.6.1 Sensation

If there are no grounds to expect sensory loss, sensation can be rapidly examined.

Briefly examine each extremity. Success depends on making the patient understand what you are doing and cooperating effectively with you. This examination is very subjective. As in the motor examination, you are looking for patterns of loss, e.g. nerve root (dermatome), nerve, sensory level (spinal cord), glove/stocking (peripheral neuropathy), dissociation (i.e. pain and temperature versus vibration and proprioception – e.g. syringomyelia).

9.8.7 Vibration Sense

- Test vibration sense using a 128 Hz tuning fork. Place the fork on the sternum first, so that the patient appreciates what vibration is. Ask the patient to close eyes, then place the vibrating fork on the lateral malleoli and wrists. Ask the patient to tell you when it stops vibrating. You stop the vibrating fork and if vibration sense is normal, the patient will tell you the vibration has stopped. If the periphery is normal, proximal sensation need not be examined. Occasionally a patient will claim to feel vibration when it is absent. If this is suspected, try a nonvibrating fork or surreptitiously stop the fork vibrating and see if the patient notices. If the patient says they can feel it vibrate, testing is not valid. Vibration sense often diminishes with age and may be absent in the legs of the elderly patient.

9.8.8 Position Sense – Proprioception

- Show the patient what you are doing. 'I am going to move your finger/toe up or down' [doing so]. 'I want you to tell me up or down each time I move it. Now close your eyes'.

- Hold distal to joint and either side with your forefinger and thumb so that pressure does not also indicate the direction of movement. Make small movements in an irregular, not alternate, sequence, e.g. up, up, down, up, down, down, down.
  Normal threshold is very low – the smallest, slowest passive movement you can produce in the terminal phalanges should always be correctly detected.

9.8.9 Pain, Touch, and Temperature

9.8.9.1 Pain and Touch

- Take a new clean neurostick/neuropin (do not reuse same neurostick/neuropin on another patient). Also take a tongue depressor.
- With the patient's eyes open touch the sharp end of the neurostick/neuropin on the skin. Do not draw blood. Ask, 'Does this feel sharp?'
- Also touch the skin with the tongue depressor. 'Does this feel blunt?'
  Ask the patient to close eyes and to tell you where you touch the skin and whether it is sharp or blunt. Then randomly assess the patient's sensory function. If you find sensory loss, map out that area by proceeding from the abnormal to normal area of skin.

9.8.9.2 Temperature

- This process can be repeated with test tubes of 'hot' (but not burning) and cold water to test perception of temperature. Ask the patient to close eyes and then tell you if they feel 'hot' or cold as you touch the skin with the test tube.

9.8.9.3 Light Touch

- Close patient's eyes.
- Ask the patient to tell you when and where you touch them with a wisp of cotton wool. Touch at irregular intervals.
- Compare both sides of body.

  Two-point discrimination. Normal threshold on fingertip is 2 mm. If sensory impairment is peripheral or in cord, a raised threshold is found, e.g. 5 mm. If cortical, no threshold is found.

  Stereognosis tested by placing coins, keys, pen top, etc. in the patient's hand and, with eyes closed, the patient attempts to identify by feeling.

  Sensory exclusion is assessed by bilateral simultaneous, e.g. touch; sensations are felt only on the normal side, whilst each is felt if applied separately. Indicates a parietal lobe lesion as brain is unable to process all stimuli.

9.8.9.4 Dermatomes

Most are easily detected with a neurostick/neuropin. Map out from area of impaired sensation.

Note in arms: middle finger – C7 and dermatomes either side symmetrical up to mid upper arm.

Note in legs: lateral border of foot and heel (S1), back of legs and anal region have sacral supply.

9.8.9.5 Gait

- Observe the patient walking. If ataxia is suspected but not seen on ordinary walking, ask the patient to do heel-to-toe walking. (Demonstrate it yourself.)

  There are many examples of abnormal gait.

- Parkinson's disease. Patient has stooped posture with most joints flexed and walks with small shuffling steps without swinging arms; tremor of hands.
- Spastic gait. Patient scrapes toe on one or both sides while walking; to prevent this the patient moves foot in a lateral arc.
- Sensory ataxia. Patient has a high stepping gait, with a slapping-down of feet. Seen with peripheral neuropathy.
- Cerebellar gait. Patient has feet wide apart while walking.
- Foot drop. Patient's toe scrapes on ground in spite of excessive lifting-up of leg on affected side.
- Shuffling gait. Patient takes multiple little steps – typical of diffuse cerebrovascular disease.
- Hysterical gait. Patient usually lurches wildly but without falling over, with the pattern marked by inconsistency.

Romberg's test is often performed at this time but is mainly a test of position sense. Ask the patient to stand upright with feet together and eyes closed. If there is any falling noted, the test is positive. Be sure you stand to the side of the patient with one arm held out in front and one arm held out to the patient's back in case the patient begins to fall so that you can steady them.

Elderly patients may fail this test and may begin to fall sideways but stop just before they topple over because of reduced proprioceptive awareness. Test positive with posterior column loss of tabes dorsalis of syphilis. Anxious patients may sway excessively; try distracting them by testing stereognosis at the same time – the excess swaying may disappear (Jarvis 2015; Swartz 2014).

9.8.10 Dorsal Column Loss of Sensation

- decreased position, vibration, and deep pain sensation (squeeze Achilles tendon)
- touch often not lost, as half carried in anterior column

9.8.11 Cortical Loss of Sensation

Defect shown by deficient function:

- position sense
- tactile discrimination
- sensory inattention

9.8.12 Signs of Meningeal Irritation

- neck rigidity – try to flex neck, is there resistance or pain?
- Kernig's sign – not as sensitive as neck rigidity.

9.8.13 Straight-Leg-Raising for Sciatica

- Lift straight leg until there is pain in back. Then slightly lower leg until there is no pain and then dorsiflex the foot to 'stretch' the sciatic nerve until the patient says there is pain present down the back of the leg.

9.9 Summary of Common Illnesses

9.9.1 Lower Motor Neuron Lesion

- wasting
- fasciculation
- hypotonia
- power diminished
- absent reflexes
- + or – sensory loss

- T1 palsy
  - weakness of the intrinsic muscles of the hand: finger adduction and abduction, thumb abduction (cf. median nerve palsy and ulnar nerve palsy)
  - sensory loss: medial forearm
- median nerve palsy
  - abductor pollicis brevis weakness (other thenar muscles may be weak) wrist drop
  - sensory loss: thumb, first 2 fingers, and palmar surface
- ulnar nerve palsy
  - interversion, hypothenar muscles wasted, weakness of finger abduction and adduction; clawhand, cannot extend fingers
  - sensory loss: half of the fourth, all of the fifth fingers, and palmar surface
- radial nerve palsy
  - wrist drop
  - sensory loss: small area/dorsal web of thumb
- L5 palsy – foot drop and weak inversion; sensory loss on medial aspect of foot
- peroneal nerve palsy – foot drop and weak eversion; minor sensory loss of dorsum of foot
- S1 palsy – cannot stand on toes, sensory loss of lateral aspect of foot, absent ankle reflex

9.9.2 Upper Motor Neuron Lesion

- no wasting
- extended arms – hand drifts down
- overswing when hands are tapped
- hypertonia
  - spastic flexion of upper limbs, extension of lower limbs
  - clasp knife
- power diminished

- increased tendon reflexes (+ or – clonus)
- extensor plantar response
- + or – sphincter disturbance
- spastic gait
    - extended stiff leg with foot drop
    - arm does not swing, held flexed

N.B. Check 'level' first, then pathology.

9.9.3 Cerebellar Dysfunction

- no wasting
- hypotonia with overswing; irregularity of movements
- intention tremor
- inability to execute rapid alternating movement smoothly (dysdiadochokinesia)
- ataxic gait
- nystagmus
- scanning or staccato speech
- incoordination not improved by sight (whereas it is with a defect of proprioception)

9.9.4 Extrapyramidal Dysfunction – Parkinson's Disease

- flexed posture of body, neck, arms, and legs
- expressionless, impassive face, staring eyes
- 'pill-rolling' tremor of hands at rest
- delay in initiating movements
- tone – 'lead pipe' rigidity, possibly with 'cog-wheeling'
- normal power and sensation
- speech quiet and monotonal
- gait – shuffling small steps, possibly with difficulty starting or stopping
- postural instability: test by having the patient standing comfortably; stand behind the patient and give a sharp tug backwards; normal patients should show a slight sway; taking steps backwards, particularly multiple steps, is abnormal

9.9.5 Multiple Sclerosis

- evidence of 'different lesions in space and time' from history and examination; usually affects cerebral white matter; common sites:
    - optic atrophy – optic neuritis
    - nystagmus – vestibular or cerebellar tracts
    - brisk jaw jerk – pyramidal lesion above fifth nerve
- cerebellar signs in arms or gait – cerebellar tracts
- upper motor neuron signs in arms or legs – pyramidal, right or left (absent superficial abdominal reflexes)
- transverse myelitis with sensory level – indicates level of lesion
- urine retention – usually sensory tract
- sensory perception loss – sensory tract

9.9.6 System-Oriented Examination

9.9.6.1 'Examine the Higher Cerebral Functions'

- general appearance
- consciousness level
- mood
- speech
- cognitive
    - confusion
    - orientation
    - attention/calculation
    - memory – short term, long term
    - reasoning – understanding of proverb

9.9.6.2 'Examine the Arms Neurologically'

- Inspect:
    - abnormal position
    - wasting
    - fasciculation
    - tremor/athetosis

- Ask patient to extend arms in front, keep them there with eyes closed, then check:
    - posture/drift
    - tap back of wrists to assess whether position is stable
    - fast finger movements (pyramidal)
    - touch nose (coordination) – finger – nose test
    - 'Hold my fingers'; push and pull against resistance
- Tone
- Muscle power – each group if indicated
- Reflexes
- Sensation
    - light touch
    - pinprick
    - vibration
    - proprioception

9.9.6.3 'Examine the Legs Neurologically'

- Inspect:
    - abnormal positions
    - wasting
    - fasciculation
- 'Lift one leg off the bed'
- 'Lift other leg off the bed'
- Coordination – heel–toe
- Tone
- Power – 'Pull up toes. Push down toes'. against resistance
- Reflexes
- Plantar reflexes
- Sensation (as hands)
- Romberg test
- Gait and tandem gait

9.9.6.4 'Examine the Arms or Legs'

- Inspect:
    - colour
    - skin/nail changes
    - ulcers
    - wasting (are both arms and legs involved?)
    - joints
- Palpate:
    - temperature, pulses
    - lumps (see above)
    - joints
        - active movements
        - feel for crepitus, e.g. hand over knee during flexion
        - passive movements (do not hurt patient)
    - reflexes
    - sensation

References

Ball, J., Dains, J., Flynn, J. et al. (2014). *Seidel's Guide to Physical Examination*, 8e. St. Louis: Elsevier Mosby.

Bickley, L. and Szilagyi, P. (2013). *Bates' Guide to Physical Examination and History Taking*, 11e. Philadelphia: Wolters Kluwer Health Lippincott Williams & Wilkins.

Boswell, G. (2004). Examination of the Nervous System in Cox, C. (Ed), *Physical Assessment for Nurses*. Oxford: Blackwell Publishing, p 121.

Crossman, A.R. and Neary, D. (2014). *Neuroanatomy: An Illustrated Colour Text*, 5e. London: Churchill Livingstone Elsevier.

Japp, A. and Robertson, C. (2013). *Macleod's Clinical Diagnosis*. Edinburgh: Churchill Livingstone, Elsevier.

Jarvis, C. (2015). *Physical Examination & Health Assessment*, 7e. St. Louis: Elsevier Saunders.

Martini, F., Nath, J., Bartholomew, E., and Petti, K. (2012). *Fundamentals of Anatomy and Physiology*, 9e. San Francisco: Benjamin Cummings.

Sirven, J. and Malamut, B. (2008). *Clinical Neurology of the Older Adult*, 2e. Wolters Kluwer Health Lippincott Williams & Wilkins.

Swartz, M. (2014). *Physical Diagnosis, History and Examination*, 7e. Philadelphia: Elsevier Saunders.

Talley, N. and O'Connor, S. (2013). *Clinical Examination: A Systematic Guide to Physical Diagnosis*, 7e. London: Churchill Livingstone Elsevier.

Tortora, G. and Derrickson, B. (2012). *Principles of Anatomy and Physiology*, 13e. Oxford: Wiley.

10 Examination of the Eye

Helen Gibbons[1,2]
[1] *Moorfields Eye Hospital NHS Foundation Trust, London, UK*
[2] *University College London, London, UK*

10.1 General Examination

10.1.1 Introduction

The purpose of examining the eye is to assess the function of the eye and its anatomy and to discern pathology that affects vision (Figure 10.1). Until recently patients with ophthalmic conditions were seen in specialist eye centres. Today more and more clinicians are assessing ophthalmic conditions in urgent care centres, emergency departments, and primary care facilities. Your assessment of the eye is important. Research has indicated that one in five people over the age of 75 live with sight loss, the main cause being age-related macular degeneration (RNIB 2015; Science Tech 2018). Many patients will be unaware that they have pathological conditions of the eye. Your assessment and intervention are essential in discerning the present and future health of a patient's eyes.

Pocket Guide to Physical Assessment, First Edition. Edited by Carol Lynn Cox.

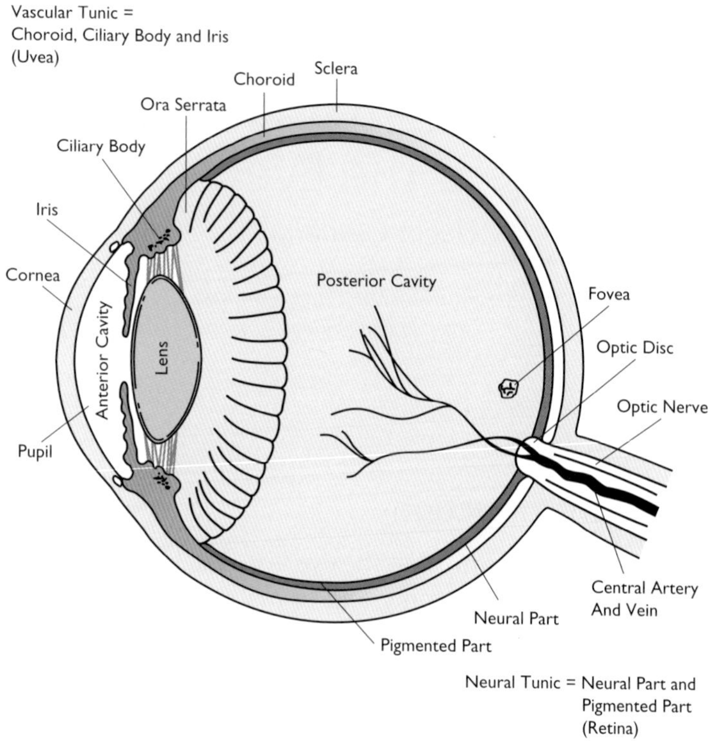

Figure 10.1 The eye. Source: Gibbons 2010. Reproduced with permission from John Wiley and Sons.

10.2 History Taking in the Ophthalmic Assessment

It is fundamentally important when examining a patient with an ophthalmic condition to have a logical and systematic approach to history taking, visual assessment, examination, and diagnosis. If this approach is not adopted, then vital signs and symptoms may be missed during the examination.

Patients with ocular symptoms often have high levels of anxiety and therefore need tact and understanding during their examination (Walsh 2006). It is therefore important to appear calm and confident in your approach Goldblum (2004) suggests that if patients are not treated in a friendly and professional manner then often they will not express all their concerns to the examiner.

In the first 2 years of life the eyeball grows rapidly. Between 10 and 13 years of age the eyeball will have reached its adult size. The scleral thickness and rigidity also increase from around 0.5 mm in childhood to 1 mm by adulthood (Wright 2003).

Children need to be treated with special care when being examined as they will often remember negative experiences which then make reexamination more traumatic, especially if they need regular follow-up. There are local anaesthetics on the market which do not smart and can be instilled before other drops that do smart to make the child's experience more comfortable.

As noted previously, it is essential to use a systematic approach in your examination and treatment of ophthalmic patients. It is good practice to:

- Take a history.
- Perform visual assessment using a Snellen Visual Acuity Chart, near vision chart, and colour vision, or Amsler Grid as required.
- Carry out a detailed examination using a good quality torch, magnifying light, and preferably a slit lamp.

The following features in the history are a requirement:

10.2.1 Presenting Complaint

- Why has the patient attended?
- Which eye is the problem (If both, did it start in one eye and transfer to the other?)

10.2.2 Duration of Symptoms

Identify:

- How long the symptoms have been present.
- Whether the symptoms are there all the time or whether they come and go.
- Whether the pain occurred suddenly or gradually.
- What the patient was doing at the time. *(Be very suspicious of penetrating injury if the patient has been drilling, chiselling, hammering, or carrying out a task that could have caused a high-speed injury.)*
- If it was a chemical injury, what it was. *(These patients need immediate irrigation with at least 1 l of normal saline, ensuring the eyelids are everted.)* Establish whether the pH of the chemical is alkaline or acid and contact the local ophthalmology unit for advice.
- If the eye has a foreign body sensation, was the patient wearing eye protection and whether the protection chosen was a good fit.
- If the patient has a discharge, it is relevant to ask whether the patient has had a recent cough or cold, as a high proportion of conjunctivitis comes from viral aetiology. Establish colour and consistency of discharge.
- Whether the patient has tried any over the counter treatments themselves at home; if yes, whether the treatments had any effect.
- If the eye has a photophobic red eye with a foreign body sensation that came on gradually, do they suffer with cold sores on their face or lip? (*It could be a Herpes simplex keratitis.)*
- If the complaint is of a headache in what region of their head is the headache positioned? Does the patient suffer with migraine? If the headache is temporal is the patient well; have they suffered weight loss, pain on touching the temporal area, or

jaw claudication? *(If yes to these questions and the patient has visual symptoms this could be temporal arteritis. Thus, the patient needs urgent bloods drawn and tested for C-reactive protein [CRP] and erythrocyte sedimentation rate [ESR] and an urgent referral to an ophthalmologist. Listen for bruits over the temporal artery as on occasion this may be heard over the temporal artery.)* If temporal pain and no visual symptoms refer to a general practitioner urgently.

- Whether the patient has any nausea and or headache. If yes, is the eye red, has a hazy cornea, and a fixed dilated pupil? *This could indicate an attack of acute glaucoma. The patient needs urgent referral to an ophthalmologist for urgent treatment.*
- Whether the patient is complaining of vision loss. Ask whether the vision is blurred. Did it worsen rapidly or over a course of weeks or months? Was it like a camera shutter closing over their eye with complete loss of vision or can they make out blurred images? Is their vision distorted when they are reading? *In sudden onset of loss of vision check blood pressure and blood sugar to exclude underlying medical conditions.*
- Whether the patient is experiencing flashing lights ± floaters; are they experiencing a cobweb or net curtain like appearance in their vision. Are they high myopes? *These patients are at higher risk of retinal detachment* (James and Bron 2011) *and require prompt referral to an ophthalmologist.*

10.2.3 Past Ocular History

Identify:

- Whether the patient has had anything similar before. If yes does the patient know what eye condition the patient had and what treatment was required?

- Whether the patient had a history of:
    - *iritis/uveitis*
    - *episcleritis/scleritis*
    - *previous eye trauma*
    - *diabetic eye disease*
    - *previous corneal abrasion/recurrent erosion syndrome*
- Whether they wear glasses for distance or reading
- *If the patient wears contact lenses, what type are they? How does the patient clean them? What is the average length of time that lenses are worn? (Overwear of contact lenses is a common cause of the red eye in contact lens wearers.)*

10.2.4 Family Ocular History

Does the patient have a history of familiar eye problems?

- *glaucoma*
- *diabetic eye disease*
- *retinal detachment*
- *diabetic eye disease*
- *squints/glasses/lazy eye*

10.2.5 General Medical Health

Do they have?

- *hypertension*
- *diabetes (how is it controlled, type and duration of symptoms)*
- *heart disease*
- *thyroid disorders*
- *joint complaints,* e.g. *rheumatoid arthritis*
- *bowel problems such as Crohn's disease*
- *chest problems such as asthma or sarcoidosis*
- *any other relevant problems*

10.2.6 Questions Relevant to Child's History Taking

Who is accompanying child?

- *parent*
- *carer*
- *sibling*
- *other relative*

What source has the referral come from?

- *school*
- *Accident and Emergency*
- *parent*

10.2.6.1 Child's Birth and Developmental Information

- *Was the child full term or premature?*
- *Was it a normal delivery, C-section or assisted,* e.g. *forceps?*
- *Does the parent have any concerns over development?*
- *Did the mother experience any problems during pregnancy,* e.g. *infections, amniocentesis?*

10.2.6.2 Other Questions Relevant to Child's History

In the young child ask the parent. In a child who can verbalise, direct the question to the child.

- *When do you notice the problem?*
  - *All the time*
  - *When tired*
  - *When unwell*

- *Is the problem getting worse?*
- *Does your child complain of headaches?*
- *Does your child bump into things?*
- *Have you noticed your child sitting close to the television?*
- *Do you sit near the board where your teacher writes?*
- *Can you see what your teacher is writing on the board?*
- *When your teacher uses different colours on the board are some colours missing?*
- *Are they frightened of the dark?*
- *Are they scared when you cover one eye?*

10.3 Allergies

Determine the allergies the patient (child, young person, adult, or older adult) has. Determine whether there are reactions the patient has when using/taking a medicine. For example, is it a food or product reaction (e.g. swelling/rash).

10.4 Occupation

- Consider what the patient's occupation is.
- Consider whether a child is at school or nursery as this may have implications for them. For example, a patient with acute bacterial or viral conjunctivitis working in a school environment or attending a nursery school needs to be advised that their condition is highly contagious, and they should refrain from work until symptoms resolve (can be anything from 24 hours to 1 week) as this can be spread to the child and staff.

10.5 Examination

10.5.1 Visual Acuity Assessment

It is an essential requirement to check and fully document a formal visual acuity. The standard assessment tool for measuring distance visual acuity is a Snellen Chart, with acuity measured at a distance of 6 m from the chart (United Kingdom Standard). *(Some charts are designed for use at shorter distances; for example, if using a reverse Snellen Chart in a mirror the vision can be measured at 3 m but still be recorded as 6 m. North American standard, 21 or 9 ft.)* The main advantage of Snellen Charts is that they are relatively straightforward to use.

10.5.2 Snellen Chart

A Snellen Chart (refer to Appendix B) is a commonly used method of measuring visual acuity. It consists of nine rows of letters that get progressively smaller. The letters are heavy block letters, numbers, or symbols printed in black on a white background. The top letter can be read by a normal eye at a distance of 60 m and the smallest line at a distance of 4 m. The vision recorded is expressed as a fraction; for example, if the patient is sitting at a distance of 6 m away from the chart and they can read the top line only then their vision in the eye being tested is 6/60. It is essential that when you record the vision you record whether the patient had their glasses or contact lenses in situ. It is not acceptable practice to record 'vision normal' or 'not affected'. If the patient is reassessed at a later date, there will not be any recordings to compare the results with, and if the patient requires referral to an eye clinic, visual acuity will be one of the first questions that will be asked.

10.5.3 Procedure

- Ensure the patient is seated comfortably with their feet firmly on the floor or footrest of the chair.
- Ask the patient to use distance glasses if needed. Test each eye individually starting with the right eye and then the left. Cover the untested eye with an occluder or a fresh tissue. (The occluder needs to be cleaned in between patients according to local policy.)
- Ask the patient to read down the chart from left to right as far as they can read. Encourage them to try another couple of letters and reassure them that it does not matter if they get a letter wrong.
- If the patient's visual acuity is anything less than 6/9 with or without glasses, it is advisable to use a pinhole to establish whether the decreased vision is correctable or not, as in some cases reduced vision is due to a refractive error and nothing more serious.
- If the patient cannot read any letters on the chart move the patient forwards 1 m closer to the chart and try the test again. If they are still unable to read the top letter, continue to move the patient forwards 1 m at a time. If at 1 m from the chart they are still unable to read the top letter, stand about 1 m away and ask the patient to count the number of fingers held up and record as counting fingers (CF). If they cannot recognise the number of fingers held up, wave your hand 30 cm in front of patient's eye and ask them if they can see your hand moving. If they can, record this as hand movements (HM). If the patient is unable to visualise HM, using your bright torch shine the light from different directions whilst asking the patient if they can see the light and which direction it is coming from. If they can see the light it can be recorded as perception to light (PL). If unable to see the light in any direction record as no perception to light (NPL).

10.5.4 The Sheridan–Gardiner Method

This test can be used in illiterate patients or in young children to obtain a Snellen Vision determination. The examiner holds a card at 6 m from the patient and asks the patient to match the letter on the corresponding card which they are holding. This gives a Snellen recording.

10.5.5 LogMAR Vision Testing

Although more complex, LogMAR vision testing is well documented as being more accurate in its measurement of visual acuity (Rosser et al. 2001). The main advantage of a LogMAR chart is that there are five letters on each line each of which is scored and therefore gives the patient a fairer chance of being able to read the letters. The main disadvantage to the tester is that it takes longer in the early stages and clinicians are put off at having to work out the scores for each individual patient. However, most departments have a conversion chart which can be used to easily record the patients score (Elliott 2007). The LogMAR vision chart is primarily used in low vision, glaucoma, and macular degeneration clinics.

10.5.6 Near Vision Testing

Near vision is assessed using a specifically designed reading card using different sizes of ordinary printer's type; each size is numbered. As in testing distance vision the patient's eyes are tested individually and using the patient's reading glasses if applicable. The chart should be used in good light, preferably with a reading light positioned over the patient's shoulder. The chart should be positioned at approximately 25 cm from the patient (Stollery 2010). Record the number of the lowest line read (e.g. N8).

10.5.7 Colour Vision Assessment

Colour vision assessment should be carried out with any patient who presents with painful loss of vision and who you suspect may have an optic nerve condition or the patient who requests a colour vision assessment for work purposes. The standard method for colour vision assessment is performed by pseudoischromatic plates such as Ishihara colour plates. These are a series of plates that test for red/green colour blindness. The plates appear as a circle of dots and within the circle a number will be placed. The patient covers one eye and reads the number. If a number on a plate cannot be distinguished a number is taken away from the total score (e.g. 16/17 read).

10.5.8 Contrast Sensitivity Testing

This test is designed to assess subtle levels of vision changes not accounted for in the normal visual acuity testing, for example, in patients with cataracts. It measures real life vision compared to black on white (Yannoff and Duker 2014). It is not routinely assessed in ophthalmology clinics but more often in research clinics. The standard chart used is a Pelli–Robson, which has six letters on each line all the same size on all eight lines. The letters fade in blackness until on the eighth row they are barely visible. Like the LogMAR test, each letter is given a score. A printed conversion sheet is provided with the Pelli–Robson chart to ensure correct interpretation of results is recorded.

10.5.9 Testing Amsler Grid

- This test is used for assessing the patient's central vision. It is an A5 sheet of paper with a grid of black lines. In the centre of the grid is a black spot.
- Each eye is tested individually. The patient needs to wear their reading glasses and holds the test at

a distance of approximately 25 cm and looks at the centre spot. They inform the examiner of any distortion, blurring, wavy or missing parts on the grid and this is then recorded on the chart. This test is of great importance in patients with suspected macular degeneration. In these cases, the patient would note wavy or distorted lines.

10.5.10 Testing Eye Movements

This test must be done in all patients who complain of double vision.

- The examiner sits in front of the patient at the same height. Explain to the patient that they must follow the pen torch with their eyes.
- Using a light from a pen torch. Ask the patient to cover their left eye and then move the light slowly up and down left and right asking the patient to report any double vision or any pain on eye movement.
- Observe for full eye movement in all directions in both eyes. Repeat the process for the other eye.

10.6 Recording Visual Fields

10.6.1 Confrontational Field Testing

- Make sure your patient is seated comfortably with their feet on the floor or footrest. You should adjust the patient's chair to ensure the patient is seated at arms-length distance from you and at eye level. You face the patient.
- Holding a large red hat pin, ask the patient to close or cover their left eye (you do the same to your opposite eye – right eye). Bring the red coloured pin into vision and ask the patient to verbalise when they can

see the pin in their visual field upper right, middle, and lower right.

- Once the right eye is examined repeat on the left eye.
- The examiner uses their observation of the pin as a guide to when the pin should come into view. Note you must have good visual fields to perform this assessment.

10.6.2 Perimetry Visual Field Testing

These tests are carried out in optometry practices and ophthalmic clinics. They measure the degree of peripheral and central visual field loss.

- They are used most frequently in glaucoma clinics to detect progression of the disease.
- The most common machine is a Humphrey field analyser. This provides an electronic record of the patient's visual field. Each eye is tested individually with the patient's refractive error corrected.
- The patient is given a buzzer to press when they see a light being shone. These lights are shone in all 360°. Recordings will show any changes to that of a normal visual field.
- The test records not only the spots correctly identified but can tell when the patient has pressed the buzzer incorrectly and whether there was any loss of fixation.

10.7 Testing the Child's Vision

There are several methods for checking a child's visual acuity. How it is performed greatly depends on the child's age and ability. Testing of a young child's visual acuity is best performed by an orthoptist in an ophthalmic unit as they are best equipped and experienced to obtain the best vision assessment from a young child. Vision in the child varies. At birth visual acuity is very poor and newborn babies are unable to fix on an object. By the age of two to four months, babies are able to fix and their vision starts to develop and will continue to do so until its peak of development at around age seven to nine years (Wright 2003).

10.7.1 Nonverbal Children

Young babies should be able to fix on a bright toy or object even if only for a few moments. By the age of six months and over the infant will try and reach out for the toy or object or pick up small sweets (small cake decorations are a useful tool for this test).

10.7.2 Verbal Children

From the age of one year there are tests specifically designed to test children's vision and these are outlined below.

10.7.3 The Cardiff Acuity Test

- This is a preferential test based on the perspective that children like to look at complex rather than plain targets.
- It is aimed at young children from about 12 months of age to 3 years of age.
- The test works by the examiner observing eye movements and response from the child to establish whether or not the child can see the target on a card.
- The cards have a grey background with a white picture. If the picture is too small for the child to see, the picture card will appear grey and the child will lose interest.
- The test is carried out at a distance of 1 m and covers vision down to 6/3.75.

10.7.4 Kay Pictures

This test is aimed at children as young as two years of age and requires the examiner to hold a series of pictures at 3 or 6 m distance.

Each card has a picture, or if using a LogMAR equivalent will have five pictures on each card getting smaller as each new card is presented. The child is asked to say what picture is on each card. If child is shy or not communicating, they can be asked to match the pictures on a corresponding card that they are holding. Once the child is of school age they can try matching the letters on a Snellen or LogMAR chart until they are able to read the letters for themselves.

10.7.5 Visual Electrophysiology Testing

In some children it is impossible to obtain a visual acuity or colour vision measurement and therefore electrophysiology in the form of an electroretinogram (ERG), visual evoked potential (VEP) and electro-oculogram (EOG) tests may be performed. These are noninvasive tests and serve as integrated parts of the ophthalmology examination. They determine how the retina and the visual cortex are functioning. These tests provide important and objective information for eye disease diagnosis, prognosis, and treatment. These tests are carried out in specialist units.

10.8 Ocular Examination of the Adult

The eye should always be examined from the outside in. When examining the patient's eye, first look at the patient's face as a whole to ensure facial symmetry and note any obvious palsy, ptosis, proptosis, or allergic reaction. Always consider the patient's age and psychological state. Patients with Parkinson's disease may, for example, find it very difficult to position themselves when a slit lamp is used to carry out the examination (Stollery 2010).

At the beginning of the examination, ask the patient to open both eyes as this is easier to do than open one alone. Use of good pen torch or magnifying light is essential (if a slit lamp is unavailable) to examine the eye and to check pupil reactions. If the patient is in pain, local anaesthetic drops may be required prior to the examination. In the case of a glass foreign body, or the history indicates a possible penetrating injury or perforation from drilling or using high-speed equipment, local anaesthetic should **not** be instilled. These patients need referral immediately to an eye unit or ophthalmic A&E (emergency) department day or night. **Do not pad the eye or put any pressure on it.** (A cartella eye shield should be used to cover the entire eye to prevent further accidental injury. A cartella eye shield is a transparent plastic shield used to protect the eye after operations.)

It is essential to look under the patient's top eyelid by everting it, if they are complaining of a foreign body sensation and a corneal foreign body cannot be seen. Use fluorescein eye drops to highlight any scratches or abrasions to the eye.

10.9 Ocular Examination of the Child

When a child attends with an eye problem requiring examination, it is essential that the child feels at ease as much as possible. Encourage young children to bring in their favourite comforter and to sit on their parent's lap if they wish. Offer the child lots of patience and reassurance. If, however, you are unsure of a diagnosis or you find a corneal foreign body, for example, contact your local eye unit for advice.

The following chart gives clear guidance on what to look for when examining eyes in both adults and children.

Face	Evaluate	■ Facial symmetry, look for drooping mouth and eyelids (Common in Bell's palsy.)
Eye movements	Can they	■ Look upwards, downwards, left, and right comfortably
	Is there	■ Any obvious squint present
Eyelids	Look for	■ Swelling of the lids *(Is the swelling hard or soft? Is it hot to touch?)* ■ Ptosis (*Droopy eyelid)* ■ Entropion *(Inturning lid)* ■ Ectropion *(Outturning lid)* ■ Trichiasis *(Ingrowing eyelashes)* ■ Any lacerations to lids ■ Chalazions ■ Blepharitis *(Inflammation to the eyelid margins)*
Conjunctiva	Assess	■ Redness *(Position and degree of redness. Is it all over? Is it localised or limbal?)* ■ Is there any haemorrhage ■ Any swelling ■ Can a foreign body be visualised ■ Is there a laceration ■ Any conjunctival cysts *(Look like a balloon filled with water.)* ■ Pterygium *(Wing-shaped growth that can encroach onto cornea causing irritation.)*
Cornea	Is it	■ Clear/hazy
	Is there	■ Any scarring ■ Staining when fluorescein dye instilled
	Are there	■ Any ulcers ■ Any foreign bodies ■ Any lacerations

Anterior chamber	Is it	■ Shallow/deep *(Compare both eyes together.)*
	Is there	■ A hyphaema *(Blood in the anterior chamber.)* ■ A hypopyon *(Pus in the anterior chamber.)* ■ Cells *(Seen when carrying out a slit lamp examination.)*
Iris	Are they	■ The same colour *(Some patients have different colour irises; some medications change the iris colour.)*
	Are there	■ Any nevus present
	Is there	■ Any trauma *(Has the patient had any previous surgery?)*
Pupil	Is it	■ Round *(A peaked pupil could indicate posterior synechiae in uveitis; an oval pupil with a hazy cornea indicates acute glaucoma.)*
	Are they	■ Equal and reactive ■ Black in colour *(In an adult a white or grey pupil often indicates a cataract; in an infant a cataract or more seriously retinoblastoma.)*

10.10 Use of a Slit Lamp

It is almost impossible to give a definite diagnosis of an eye condition without using a slit lamp.

- The slit lamp consists of a microscope and a light source.
- Slit lamp examination is indicated in any condition of the eyelids or eyeball. Ocular conditions can be better diagnosed and treated by having a highly illuminated, magnified view.

Technique

- Explain to patient that the light may be a little bright but that it will give a highly magnified view of the eye; thus, aiding diagnosis.
- Patient and examiner are seated (both must be comfortable) with the patient chin height adjusted, to ensure the eye is aligned with the slit lamp guide.
- Patient places chin and forehead on bars; examiner looks through the eyepieces (The examiner has adjusted the eyepieces to their own glasses prescription.)
- The lids, cornea, anterior chamber, and iris can be easily viewed by moving the focus from the joystick, forwards and backwards as required.
- Use fluorescein and the blue cobalt light to look for corneal staining and corneal abrasions.
- Use slit beam, approximately 1 mm wide and 3 mm long with high magnification to look for anterior chamber cells and flare.

10.10.1 The Use of a 90 Dioptre Lens with a Slit Lamp to View the Retina

This examination is usually carried out in optometry practices and hospital clinics. Extra training should be undertaken prior to carrying out this procedure. It gives a much better view of the retina than direct ophthalmoscopy and is therefore used more in the hospital setting than a direct ophthalmoscope.

- This procedure can be carried out with an undilated pupil; however, a better image will be seen through a dilated pupil.
- Ensure the 90 D lens is clean and smear free. (Clean only with a lens cloth to prevent scratching on the lens coating.)

- Ensure that the patient is comfortably and correctly positioned at the slit lamp with their chin on the chin rest, forehead firmly pressed against the plastic strap, head pointing straight ahead, and patient's eye in line with the mark on the metal frame of the slit lamp.
- Adjust the power of the light so that it is not too bright for the patient. Adjust the width of the slit so that it is 2–3 mm wide and the height of the beam to about 8 mm.
- Pull the slit lamp joystick towards you
- To examine the patient's right eye, hold the 90 D lens in your left hand.
- Ask the patient to look at your right ear or use the fixation light.
- Hold the 90 D lens just in front of the patient's right eye without touching the eye with the lens. Hold the lens with the thumb and index finger.
- Using your right hand, slowly advance the slit lamp towards the eye. At first the lens will be seen with an inverted image of the eye in its centre. (The image is vertically and laterally inverted and virtual.)

10.10.2 Fundus Examination

- As the slit lamp is moved closer to the patient, the vitreous and then the retina should come into view. With the patient looking in the direction you tell them to, the disc should come into view. From the nasal side to the disc, the macula can be seen. Examine the retinal vessels for any signs of haemorrhages or occlusion.
- To examine the temporal retina, ask the patient to look to their right.
- To examine the nasal retina, ask the patient to look to their left.

- Get the patient to look up for the superior retina, then down for the inferior retina. The patient's upper lid will need to be kept open by gently lifting it with a finger when the patient looks down.
- The image seen in all directions of gaze is vertically and laterally inverted. For example, on up gaze, the superior most part of the retina is in the inferior field. This must be remembered when drawing the image, but a useful tip is to turn the page upside down; thus, you can draw what you are seeing and on turning the page round the image will be presented correctly.
- Repeat the entire process to examine the patient's left fundus; this time using your right hand to hold the lens, with the patient looking at your left ear, to see the disc.

10.11 Measurement of Intraocular Pressure

This test is carried out on most patients who attend an ophthalmology clinic and on all patients who are over the age of 40 in optometry practices. The usual intraocular eye pressure is between 10 and 21 mmHg (Coakes and Holmes 1995)

10.11.1 Goldmann Tonometry

- The gold standard method is by Goldmann tonometry. This provides the most accurate measurement, but it is difficult to master and should be carried out only after specialist training.
- Fluorescein dye and anaesthetic dye is instilled in the eye.
- A clear plastic prism is advanced until it touches the cornea. Two semicircles are seen, and the two inner

circles meet. The measurement can then be read on the dial at the side of the instrument.

10.11.2 Perkins Applanation Tonometry

- This is a handheld device useful for patients unable to be seen on a slit lamp.
- It has the same principles as Goldmann tonometry.
- It is difficult to master.
- In order to obtain this measurement, the examiner needs to get very close to patient.

10.11.3 Tonopen

- This is easy to use and is good for emergency departments and patients who are unable to reach a slit lamp.
- It is a penlike device which when gently tapped on an anaesthetised cornea will give you an intraocular pressure (IOP) reading.

10.11.4 Air Puff

- Most commonly used in optometry practices.
- Can give abnormally high readings as it makes the patient jump or hold their breath.
- The time taken to flatten the cornea is converted into a figure to give an IOP.

10.12 Palpation of the Globe

- Palpation of the eye using two fingers on a closed eyelid with the patient looking downwards.
- Is of no value other than to detect the hardness in an acute glaucoma (Coakes and Holmes 1995).

10.13 Use of an Ophthalmoscope

- Make sure that the ophthalmoscope is fully charged and has a bright light and the bulb is in working order before the examination commences.
- The patient should be sitting. Remove spectacles from yourself and the patient.
- Begin by setting the lens dioptre dial at 0 if you do not use spectacles. If you are myopic, you should start with the 'minus' lenses. Set the lens dioptre at −4 to begin, which is indicated as a red number. If you are hyperopic you should use the 'plus' lenses, which are indicated by black numbers. Keep your index finger on the dial to permit easy focusing. Hold the ophthalmoscope about 30 cm from the patient. Shine the light into the patient's pupil, identify the red reflex (from the retina), and approach the patient at an angle of 15°. Approach on the same horizontal plane as the equator of the patient's eye. This will bring you straight to the patient's optic disc. After observing the disc examine the peripheral retina fully by following the blood vessels to and back from the four main quadrants.
- Hold the ophthalmoscope in your right hand in front of your right eye to examine the patient's right eye, and in your left hand in front of your left eye to examine the patient's left eye. Try to hold your breath when using the ophthalmoscope. Do not breathe into the patient's face.
- If the patient's pupils are small, dilate with 1% tropicamide, one drop per eye. Tropicamide works in 15–20 minutes and lasts 2–4 hours. Warn the patient that their vision will be blurred for approximately 4 hours. Do **not** dilate if neurological observation of pupils is needed.

- The patient should be told they cannot drive, if their pupils have been dilated, for at least 4–6 hours.

10.13.1 Look at Optic Disc

- normally pink rim with white 'cup' below surface of disc
- *optic atrophy*
  - disc pale: rim no longer pink
  - *multiple sclerosis*
  - *after optic neuritis*
  - *optic nerve compression*, e.g. *tumour*
  - papilloedema
  - *disc pink, indistinct margin*
  - *cup disappears*
  - *dilated retinal veins*
  - *increased cerebral pressure*, e.g. *tumour*
  - *accelerated hypertension*
  - *optic neuritis, acute stage*
  - glaucoma – enlarged cup, diminished rim
  - new vessels – new fronds of vessels coming forwards from disc
  - ischaemic *diabetic retinopathy*

10.13.2 Look at Arteries

- arteries narrowed in hypertension, with increased light reflex along top of vessel

1. Hypertension grading:
2. narrow arteries
3. 'nipping' (narrowing of veins by arteries)
4. flame-shaped haemorrhages and cotton-wool spots
5. papilloedema

- occlusion artery – pale retina
- occlusion vein – haemorrhages

10.13.3 Look at Retina

- hard exudates (shiny, yellow circumscribed patches of lipid)
  - *diabetes*
- cotton-wool spots (soft, fluffy white patches)
  - microinfarcts causing local swelling of nerve fibres
    - *diabetes*
    - *hypertension*
    - *vasculitis*
    - *human immunodeficiency virus* (HIV)
- small, red dots
  - microaneurysms – retinal capillary expansion adjacent to capillary closure
    - *diabetes*
- haemorrhages
  - round ‘blots’: haemorrhages deep in retina larger than microaneurysms
    - *diabetes*
  - flame shaped: superficial haemorrhages along nerve fibres
    - *hypertension*
    - *gross anaemia*
    - *hyperviscosity*
    - *bleeding tendency*
  - Roth’s spots (white-centred haemorrhages)
    - *microembolic disorder*
    - *subacute bacterial endocarditis*
- pigmentation
  - widespread
    - *retinitis pigmentosa*
  - localised

choroiditis (clumping of pigment into patches)
drug toxicity, e.g. chloroquine

- tigroid or tabby fundus: normal variant in choroid beneath retina

- peripheral new vessels
  ischaemic diabetic retinopathy
  retinal vein occlusion
- medullated nerve fibres – normal variant, areas of white nerves radiating from optic disc

10.14 Pupil Assessment for Relative Afferent Papillary Defect (RAPD)

This is an essential test to perform prior to dilating drops being instilled, especially in patients who you suspect have optic nerve conditions.

- Assess size and shape of pupils
- Sit the patient in a dimly lit room
- Ask the patient to gaze into the distance
- Shine the bright torch from one eye to the other (hold light on pupil for two to three seconds on each eye); if there is a pupil defect the pupil will dilate instead of constricting when the eye is illuminated. The normal response would be for the pupil to constrict when the light is shone on pupil.

10.15 Documentation

When documenting your findings, it is essential to document in a systematic format. An example is outlined below.

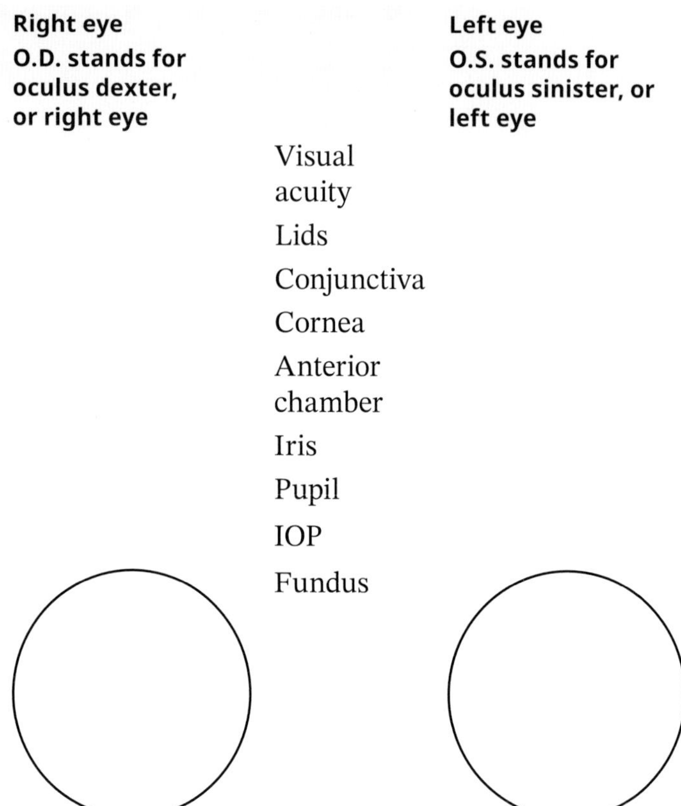

Corneal topography is also known as photokeratoscopy or videokeratography. It is a noninvasive medical imaging technique for mapping the surface curvature of the cornea, which is the outer structure of the eye. Its topography is of critical importance in determining the quality of vision and corneal health because the cornea is responsible for approximately 70% of the eye's refractive power.

Phoropter is an ophthalmic testing device that is also called a refractor. It contains different lenses used for refraction of the eye during sight testing. It measures a person's refractive error and determines the spectacle prescription.

References

Coakes, R. and Holmes, S. (1995). *Outline of Ophthalmology*, 2e. Oxford: Butterworth Heineman.

Elliott, D. (2007). *Clinical Procedures in Primary Eye Care*, 3e. Edinburgh: Butterworth Heineman.

Gibbons, H. (2010) Ophthalmic Examination, in Cox, C. (ed), *Physical Assessment for nurses, 2e.* Oxford: Wiley Blackwell pp 181–203.

Goldblum, K. (2004). Obtaining a complete and pertinent patient history. *Insight / American Society of Ophthalmic Registered Nurses, Inc.* XXIX (2): 17–20. April–June.

James, B. and Bron, A. (2011). *Lecture Notes on Ophthalmology*, 11e. Oxford: Wiley-Blackwell Publishing.

RNIB (2015) www.rnib.co.uk (accessed 30 December 2015).

Rosser, D., Laidlaw, D., and Murdoch, I. (2001). The development of a "reduced LogMAR" visual acuity chart for use in routine clinical practice. *British Journal of Ophthalmology* 85: 432–436.

Science Tech (2018) Stem Cell Discovery In Eyes Could Possibly Be Used To Cure Age-Related Blindness

Stollery, R. (2010). *Ophthalmic Nursing*, 4e. Oxford: Wiley-Blackwell Publishing.

Walsh, M. (2006). *Nurse Practitioners: Clinical Skills and Professional Issues*, 2e. Edinburgh: Elsevier.

Wright, K. (2003). *Paediatric Ophthalmology for Primary Care*, 2e. Edinburgh: Elsevier.

Yannoff, M. and Duker, J. (2014). *Ophthalmology*, 4e. London: Mosby.

11 Examination of the Musculoskeletal System

Nicola L. Whiteing
Southern Cross University, New South Wales, Australia

11.1 General Examination

11.1.1 Introduction

The musculoskeletal assessment constitutes an essential aspect in evaluating the patient's health. Functions of the musculoskeletal system involve a functional relationship between the muscles and bones of the body (Martini et al. 2012). Changes in the musculoskeletal system affect other systems.

11.1.1.1 Assessment/Examination

Musculoskeletal disorders are common and major causes of ill health accounting for over 21 million general practitioner consultations alone in the United Kingdom in 2015 (MKS Toolkit 2015) and 50% (126 million in ages 18 and over) of primary care consultations in the United States of America in 2014 (Bone and Joint Initiative 2014). In Europe, musculoskeletal conditions are the most common cause of severe long-term pain and disability (22%) (EU Report v5.0 2010). Musculoskeletal conditions lead to significant healthcare and social support costs and are a major cause of work absence and incapacity. In addition, they have a significant

Pocket Guide to Physical Assessment, First Edition. Edited by Carol Lynn Cox.

economic cost through lost productivity and can seriously affect the quality of life of those with the conditions and of their families, friends, and carers (EU Report v5.0 2010).

For the patient presenting with a musculoskeletal problem, the primary complaint is likely to be that of pain or a decrease in functional ability. These are symptoms that the patient is unlikely to ignore. Therefore, musculoskeletal complaints make up a large amount of the primary care or minor injury practitioner's caseload. The aim of the musculoskeletal assessment is to determine the degree to which the patient's activities of living are affected, through a systematic assessment. The musculoskeletal assessment is closely linked with the neurological assessment as bone and muscle functioning is directly coordinated by the central nervous system (Ball et al. 2014a, b; Barkauskas et al. 2002; Bickley and Szilagyi 2007, 2013; Dains et al. 2012, 2015; Epstein et al. 2008). You should read the neurological assessment in Chapter 9 in conjunction with this chapter.

11.2 Frequent Musculoskeletal Complaints

11.2.1 Sprains and Strains

Sprains and strains are the most common musculoskeletal complaint the practitioner might encounter in either urgent care, a primary care setting, or minor injury unit. Careful consideration must be given when using above terms to convey the exact nature of injury. Strain refers to an injury of tendons or tearing of muscle fibres as a result of overstretching. Sprain, on the other hand, refers to ligamental injuries resulting from overstretching a unit over its functional range of movement (ROM; Ball et al. 2014a, b; Bickley and Szilagyi 2007, 2013; Dains et al. 2012, 2015; Japp and Robertson 2013; Jarvis 2008, 2015; Seidel et al. 2006, 2010; Swartz 2006, 2014; Talley and O'Connor 2006, 2014; Tallia and Scherger 2013).

11.2.2 Osteoarthritis

A degenerative joint disease due to a progressive breakdown of the joint surfaces. Direct and indirect trauma to the articular cartilage and infection can all lead to osteoarthritis. Osteoarthritis primarily affects weight-bearing joints (hips, knees) with patients presenting to their medical provider with increased pain and a decrease in their functional ability. The end result is often a joint replacement. However, symptoms can often be managed/ reduced through a range of pharmacological and nonpharmacological means.

11.2.3 Rheumatoid Arthritis

This is the most common chronic inflammatory disease of joints. A systemic disease causing many different structures to be affected. Unlike osteoarthritis, which invariably affects one joint in isolation, treatment aims to control the pain associated with synovitis and maintain as much function as possible.

11.2.4 Osteoporosis

Because of a lack of oestrogen in postmenopausal women, a reduction in the amount of collagen in bones occurs. The bone becomes thin and a kyphosis of the spine is often seen with pain over the spinous processes. Fractures of the femoral neck and crush fractures of the vertebrae are common after a minor trip or fall.

11.2.5 Fractures

Fractures are usually caused by trauma either significant, or minor and repeated. Pathological fractures occur as a result of disease, e.g. tumours, osteoporosis, Paget's disease, and osteomalacia. There are many types of fracture. However, the principles behind their management remain the same.

11.3 Key Principles of Musculoskeletal Assessment

- Consider the nature of presenting complaint to align and focus your assessment bearing in mind other systemic causes. In general, the nature of the presenting complaint could be pain, swelling, crepitus, locking, wasting, fasciculation, or cramps.
- The nature of symptom onset whether trauma related, insidious, or episodic is vital in establishing severity.
- The ROM and limiting factors will establish effects on activities of living.
- Ascertain possible nonmusculoskeletal origin of pain including referred pain.

11.4 Practical Considerations

- In order that a comprehensive musculoskeletal assessment is undertaken, the patient will have to be exposed.
- The patient should be allowed to re-dress as the examination proceeds or be covered as appropriate to ensure privacy and dignity.
- The musculoskeletal assessment has two stages: inspection and palpation. Unlike other systems examinations, you should work through the two stages together rather than inspecting all joints and then returning to palpate.
- Always ask whether the patient has any pain and if so, assess the pain-free side first.
- Arrange your assessment by examining each area in relation to patient comfort, allowing the joint/extremity to be supported.
- Always compare each side.
- Organise your examination of the bones, muscles, and joints in a head-to-toe method. This will help avoid omissions.

- Certain situations will require you to perform a movement so the patient can emulate.
- Always start each part of the examination from the neutral position.

11.5 Assessment Consideration

Your assessment should seek to elicit the source and tissue type involved in the presentation. The two tissue types for consideration are:

- Inert tissues: bone, cartilage, capsule, ligaments, and bursa
- Contractile tissues: muscle, musculotendinous junction, body of tendon, bone at insertion of tendon.

Different assessment techniques are required for the type of tissue involved in the presentation (see ROMs below).

11.6 Legal Consideration

Because of the increasing litigation culture careful consideration should be given to any potential litigation following musculoskeletal assessment. With this in mind, the traditional assessment of look, feel, and move can be modified in suspicious circumstances. It is important at times to consider and document limitations of active movements by the patient prior to any passive movement or manipulation by the practitioner (Thomas and Monaghan 2007; Walsh 2006).

11.7 Inspection

For a comprehensive assessment, inspection should commence as patient walks into consulting room observing for gait and body alignment. Inspection should be carried out observing from anterior, posterior, and lateral views. Inspection should assess for:

- size
- contour
- symmetry
- involuntary movements (tremors, fasciculations)
- deformities (subluxation, dislocation, varus, valgus)
- swelling/oedema (effusions, haematoma)
- discolouration (vascular insufficiency, bruising, haematoma)
- hypertrophy/atrophy of muscles (steroid use, malnutrition, spinal cord lesion)
- posture and body alignment
- structural relationships
- scars indicating any previous surgery or trauma
- condition of skin (pressure ulcers, necrosis, scarring)

11.8 Palpation

- Palpate joints, bursal sites, bones, and surrounding muscles.
- Assess the patient for both verbal and nonverbal cues of pain.
- Ask the patient, 'Does the pain radiate elsewhere from the initial region?'
- Palpation should assess for the following:
    - increased temperature (use the back of the hand above, below, and on the joint and compare with the other side)
    - swelling/oedema
    - tenderness
    - crepitus (loose cartilage [etc.], listen for crepitus as well as feeling)
    - consistency and tone of muscle

11.9 Range of Movement

- Assess the degree of deviation away from the neutral position.
- A goniometer should be used to obtain an accurate ROM (Japp and Robertson 2013; Jarvis 2008, 2015).
    - Active ROM involves the patient moving the joint himself. Active movements test:
        - Inert and contractile tissues
        - Test for pain, power, and range
    - Movement should be smooth and pain free.
    - Passive ROM involves you providing motion in order to move the joint. Passive movements:
        - Test inert (eliminates muscle, tendon, and tenoperiosteal junction)
        - Test for pain, range, and feel
        - Test for passive stretch or squeezing
- Resisted involves the practitioner initiating the movement with the patient opposing the movement. Resisted movement:
    - Test contractile tissues if no movement of joint, e.g. 'I am going to push foot up; don't let me'
    - Assess for pain and weakness
    - Isometric contraction
    - Stress testing involves:
    - Passive stretching of ligaments to detect injury

Question whether:

- Active ROM is less than passive ROM – focus on true weakness, joint stability, pain, and malignancy.
- Active and passive ROM is limited – determine whether there is any excess fluid or any loose bodies in the joint (e.g. cartilage), joint surface irregularity (e.g. osteoarthritis, contracture of muscle, ligaments, or capsule).

11.10 Limb Measurement

- Ensure limbs are in the neutral position.
- Ensure the patient is lying straight – many discrepancies in limb length are due to inaccurate positioning.
- Full length upper limb – measure from the acromion process to the end of the middle finger.
- Upper arm only – acromion process to the olecranon process.
- Lower arm only – olecranon process to the styloid process of the ulna.
- Full length lower limb – lower edge of the ileum to tibial malleolus.
- Upper leg only – lower edge of the ileum to the medial aspect of the knee.
- Lower leg only – medial aspect of the knee to the tibial malleolus.

  Establish whether shortening is due to a loss of bone length or a deformity at the joint, e.g. a hip dislocation.

11.11 Bones

Examine for:

- deformity
- tumours
  - pain – is the pain focal (fracture/trauma, infection, malignancy, Paget's disease, osteoid osteoma), or diffuse (malignancy, Paget's disease, osteomalacia, osteoporosis, metabolic bone disease)?
  - consider character, onset, site, radiation, severity, periodicity, exacerbating, and relieving factors, diurnal variation.

11.12 Joints

Always compare each joint bilaterally to make a comparison. Examine for:

- pain – causes include inflammatory (e.g. rheumatoid arthritis), mechanical (e.g. osteoarthritis), infective (e.g. pyogenic tuberculosis), or traumatic (e.g. fractures).
- questions to ask:
  - Where is the maximal site of pain?
  - Does the pain change during the course of the day?
  - Has the pain been there for a short or long time?
  - Does the pain get better or worse as the patient moves about?
- tenderness
- swelling
- partial or complete loss of mobility
- stiffness
- deformity
- weakness
- fatigue
- warmth
- redness
- lesions or ulcers

Pitting of nails is present in 50% of cases of joint disease.

11.13 Muscles

Assess:

- size
- contour

- tone
- strength/weakness
    - questions to ask:
        - Is the weakness global or focal?
        - Is the weakness secondary to a painful limb?
        - Does the weakness fluctuate in degree?
        - Is the weakness increasing in severity?
        - Is the weakness associated with sensory symptoms or signs?
        - Is there a family history of muscle disease?
        - Is the weakness symmetrical?
        - Is the weakness predominantly proximal or distal?
- pain – causes include inflammatory (e.g. polymyalgia rheumatica), infective (e.g. pyogenic cysticercosis), traumatic, or neuropathic (e.g. Guillain–Barré syndrome).

11.14 The Examination

When asking the patient to perform active ROM, instruct them in a way that will be understood. It may be necessary for you to perform the movement first so that the patient can then copy it.

11.15 Gait, Arms, Legs, Spine Screen

The gait, arms, legs, spine (GALS) screen provides a useful rapid screen of the overall integrity of the locomotor system. It is felt that the general survey (described next) followed by a regional joint examination is necessary for the patient presenting with a musculoskeletal complaint; however, the GALS screen may be used to make a quick 'screening' examination of the whole locomotor system in order to identify an abnormality in the absence of symptoms (Doherty et al. 1992; Thomas and Monaghan 2007).

11.16 General Survey

The general survey should start as soon as you meet the patient. Call the patient into the examination room and look at how they move. You can gain an accurate assessment of the patient's pattern of gait as they enter the room – once you ask the patient to walk for you the gait may change. Watch the patient throughout the examination. Observe how they get on and off the examination couch and up from a chair. Look at the speed of manoeuvres and any pain elicited.

Shake the patient's hand and gain an idea of muscle strength.

Observe the patient's gait anteriorly and posteriorly, with and without shoes on:

- Does the patient trip?
- Is there a limp present? – Look at the patient's shoes and see if one side of the heel is worn more than the other.
- Alignment of the pelvis and shoulders during walking.
- Does the patient stagger to one particular side?
- Does the patient, despite apparently severe ataxia, seldom sustain injury?
- If a Trendelenburg gait pattern is suspected, ask the patient to stand on one leg; if the hip abductors are weak, the pelvis will tilt towards the non-weight-bearing side.
- For examples of abnormal gait patterns, refer to Chapter 11.

General inspection:

- Posture
- Body alignment
- Hypertrophy/atrophy of the muscles – dominant side is usually slightly bigger than the nondominant. Hypertrophy can be seen in young men using steroids. Atrophy of the muscles can be due to malnutrition, lack of use of muscles due to joint disease, or a spinal cord lesion due to the lack of neural input to the muscle. May need to measure the circumference of muscle bulk and document on each visit to assess any decrease. Differences of <1 cm noted at different times are not significant.
- Genu valgum/genu varum
- Hyperextension of the knees – will often indicate hypermobility of all joints; however, hypermobility could be due to ligament ruptures, intraarticular fractures, or connective tissue disruption, e.g. Marfan's syndrome.
- Carrying angle – elbows should be at approximately 5–15° in an adult.
- Spine – scoliosis, kyphosis, lordosis, gibbus
- Symmetry
- Contour
- Size
- Involuntary movements
- Gross deformities
- Limb measurement

11.17 Regional Examination

11.17.1 Jaw

The temporomandibular joint (TMJ) – the articulation between the temporal bone and the mandible.

- Place fingertips over the TMJ, anterior to the external meatus of the ear.
- Palpate whilst the patient goes through the ROMs:
    - open and close the mouth – extension
    - project the lower jaw – flexion
    - move the jaw from side to side – abduction and adduction
    - is there any crepitus?
- Ask the patient to bite down hard – palpate the muscle strength of the masseter muscles.
- Ask the patient to clench teeth whilst you push lightly on the chin – also tests the motor function of cranial nerve V.

11.17.2 Spine

- Normal curvatures at the spine are concave at the cervical region, convex at the thoracic region, and concave at the lumbar region.

11.17.3 I Cervical Spine

The sternoclavicular joint – the articulation between the sternum and the clavicle.

The cervical vertebrae – C1–C7, most mobile of all spinal vertebrae.

- Using thumbs, palpate all spinous processes.
- Palpate along the clavicles and manubrium of the sternum.
- Observe patient going through the ROMs:
    - chin to chest – flexion
    - raise the head back to the neutral position – extension
    - bend the head backwards – hyperextension
    - turn head to each side – lateral rotation
    - place each ear to each shoulder – lateral bending

- To test the muscle strength of the trapezius and sternocleidomastoid muscles, the above ROMs should be performed to resistance.

11.17.4 II Thoracic and Lumbar Spine

Thoracic vertebrae – T1–T12.
Lumbar vertebrae – L1–L5.

- Look at equality of height at the shoulders and the iliac crests.
- Using your thumbs, palpate along all spinous processes – if no pain is elicited, but malignancy or osteoporosis is suspected, light percussion of the spinous processes using the ulnar aspect of your fist may prove a useful technique.
- Palpate around the scapulae and assess for equality in height.
- Have the patient stand with feet 15 cm apart and ask them to bend forwards slowly as if touching toes. Observe for any abnormal curvatures of the spine:
    - scoliosis – a lateral curvature of the spine
    - lordosis – an exaggerated lumbar curvature (can be normal during pregnancy, in the obese or women of Afro-Caribbean origin)
    - kyphosis – a rounded thoracic convexity (commonly known as the 'Dowager's hump'); common in osteoporotic women
    - gibbus – when a defect is of a sharp angle, the spinous processes are seen more prominently on the back forming an apex
    - list – the spine is tilted to one side with no compensation
- If the patient is able to stay in a flexed position, it is useful for you to palpate the patient's spinous processes whilst in this position. An early scoliosis

may be detected through palpation, which may be missed upon inspection in the upright position.

- A spinal curvature may have an effect on the patient's respiratory function, thus, attention may also need to be paid to a respiratory assessment.
- Observe the patient going through the ROMs:
    - Bend forwards to touch toes – flexion.
    - Stand back up into the neutral position – extension.
    - Bend back as far as possible running hands down the back of the thighs – hyperextension.
    - Run a hand down each leg laterally – lateral bending.
    - Turn to the right and left in a circular motion – rotation*.

  It is important that you stabilise the patient's pelvis during this ROM, or the movement will come from the pelvis and not the spine. You should have the patient sitting in a chair or on an examination couch/table with arms crossed to assess this movement.
- To assess the muscle strength of the trapezius and paravertebral muscles, the above should be performed to resistance.

11.17.4.1 Stretch Tests

- If a patient presents with a history of lower back pain, you should assess ability to straight leg raise (SLR) with the Lasegue Test. If Lasegue Test is positive then the Bragard test should be included as an extra manoeuvre.
    - The patient should lie supine with the leg as relaxed as possible. You should slowly raise the

---

*Internal rotation or medial rotation and external rotation or lateral rotation

foot, keeping the knee straight until the patient complains of pain, then dorsiflex the foot.

  - You should make a note of the ROM obtained before a complaint of pain and whether the pain intensifies upon dorsiflexion of the foot.
  - A positive SLR test includes pain before 70° is reached in an L5 or S1 distribution, increased pain on dorsiflexion of the foot along the sciatic nerve trajectory, and relief of pain on flexion of the knee (Barkauskas et al. 2002; Seidel et al. 2006, 2010; Walsh 2006).
  - A positive test is indicative of a herniated lumbar disc.
- If it is felt that a lumbar disc may have prolapsed higher (L2–L4) a stretch test for the femoral nerve should be performed.
  - The patient should lie prone and extend the hip with the knee in a flexed position.
  - Note the point at which the patient complains of pain.
  - Pain will be elicited in the lumbar region as the femoral nerve roots are tightened.
  - Lying prone may not be possible for all patients, so an alternative test can be performed with the patient lying laterally with knees bent. This position produces a stretch of the femoral nerve. The stretch is enhanced as the patient bends the head towards the chest.
- Patella and Achilles reflexes should also be tested.

11.17.5 Upper Limb

11.17.5.1 Shoulder

The acromioclavicular joint – the articulation between the acromion process of the scapula and the clavicle.

The glenohumeral joint – the articulation between the glenoid fossa and the humerus.

The sternoclavicular joint – the articulation between the sternum and the clavicle.

- Inspect the shoulder from anterior and posterior views.
- Look at the shape of the shoulders – anterior dislocation of the shoulder can be seen as a flattening of the lateral aspect. Check for altered sensation laterally as the axillary nerve may have been damaged by the dislocation.
- Look for swelling at the joint.
- Observe the equality of shoulder height.
- Look for muscle wasting – may be present in arthritic joints when the patient does not use the arm.
- Palpate each of the shoulder joints and the bursal sites (subacromial bursa and subscapular bursa).
- Assess the temperature of the joint and note any colour changes in conjunction with an increased temperature.
- Palpate the clavicles, scapulae, acromion process and biceps groove.
- Palpate the associated muscles – particularly those of the rotator cuff.
- Observe the patient going through the ROM:
    - extend both arms forwards – flexion
    - back to the neutral position – extension
    - extend both arms backwards – hyperextension
    - put an arm out to the side – abduction
    - put an arm across the body – adduction
    - roll arms forwards and backwards in a circular motion – circumduction
    - put an arm behind the back and touch the opposite shoulder blade – internal rotation

- put an arm behind the head – external rotation
- draw shoulders upwards – elevation
- draw the shoulders downwards – depression
- draw the shoulders forwards – protraction
- draw the shoulder back – retraction – gives a good view of the equality of scapula height.

11.17.5.2 Elbow

The articulation between the humerus, radius, and ulna.

- Inspect and palpate with the elbow in a flexed and extended position.
- Inspect for swelling, redness, and increased temperature.
- Inspect for tracking marks and any associated cellulitis in the cubital fossa region – drug misuse.
- Palpate the olecranon bursa, the distal humerus, medial and lateral epicondyles, the olecranon process, coronoid process of the ulna and the radius.
- Assess for any pain or tenderness over the annular ligament.
- Assess for any joint swelling in the grooves either side of the olecranon process.
- Observe the patient going through the ROM:
    - bend the arm – flexion
    - straighten the arm – extension
    - turn the hand palm up – supination
    - turn the hand palm down – pronation

    Ensure that the elbow is flexed to 90° and is locked against the side of the body when testing supination and pronation; otherwise the movement will come from the glenohumeral joint and not that of the elbow.

11.17.5.3 Wrist

The articulation between the distal radius and the proximal portions of the carpus.

- Inspect both wrists for symmetry, contour, swelling, atrophy, and smoothness.
- Because of little tissue covering the dorsal aspect of the wrist joint, swelling is clearly visible.
- Use thumbs and index fingers to palpate the wrist and proximal portions of the carpus.
- Apply pressure in the anatomical snuff box – fractures of the scaphoid are not clearly visible on plain A–P and lateral X-rays and scaphoid views are needed. Pain in the anatomical snuff box is a good indicator of a fracture. If not diagnosed and treated quickly, the patient is at risk of avascular necrosis, particularly if the fracture is through the highly vascular proximal pole.
- Palpate the ulna tip for any pain and across the underlying bones of the carpus – scaphoid, lunate, pisiform, trapezium, trapezoid, hamate, and capitate.
- Observe the patient going through the ROMs:
    - bend hand down – flexion
    - bend hand upwards – extension
    - with the hand pronated, turn it towards the right – radial deviation
    - with the hand pronated, turn it towards the left – ulna deviation
- If carpal tunnel syndrome is suspected, one of two tests can be carried out:
    - Phalen's test – ask the patient to maintain palmar flexion for one minute. This will produce numbness. When hands are brought back to the normal position the numbness disappears.
    - Tinel's test – lightly tap the median nerve. This will produce a tingling which will stop when tapping is ceased.

11.17.5.4 Fingers

Metacarpophalangeal joints – the articulation between the distal portions of the carpus and the metacarpal bones.

Proximal interphalangeal joints – the articulation between the metacarpal and the proximal phalanges.

Distal interphalangeal joints – the articulation between the proximal and distal phalanges.

- Inspect each of the fingers and each of the joints – rheumatoid arthritis is particularly evident in the joints of the fingers.
- Look at the condition of the nails.
- Using the thumb and index finger, palpate each of the metacarpophalangeal and interphalangeal joints.
- Observe the patient going through the ROMs:
  - make a fist – full finger flexion
  - open a fist – full finger extension
  - spread fingers out – abduction
  - bring fingers in together from abduction – adduction
  - push fingers forwards – hyperflexion
  - push fingers backwards – hyperextension
  - little finger to thumb – opposition
  - thumb to little finger – opposition
- Carry out ROM with wrist flexed as well as in neutral to test for tendon shortening.

11.17.6 Lower Limb

11.17.6.1 Pelvis and Hips

The sacroiliac joints – the articulation between the sacrum and the ileum.

The symphysis pubis – The articulation bilaterally between the inferior and superior pubic rami.

The hip joint – the articulation between the acetabulum and the femur.

- Inspect the iliac crests for symmetry and equality of height.
- Look at the number and level of gluteal folds.
- Look at the size of the buttocks.
- Inspect the femoral area for signs of tracking and associated cellulitis – drug misuse.
- In supine position, inspect the body alignment looking for external rotation of the hips and inequality of leg length – often seen in osteoarthritis, fractures, or dislocations of the hip.
- Gait – (refer to the general survey in this chapter and Chapters 3 and 11).
- Palpate bursal sites.
- In supine position, palpate hips and pelvis for tenderness, increased temperature, or crepitus.
- Rock the pelvis from side to side whilst holding the iliac crests to test for stability at the sacroiliac joints.
- With the patient lying prone, apply slight pressure to the sacrum to test for stability at the symphysis pubis – this joint can become lax in women carrying and/or following the birth of large babies.
- Observe the patient going through the ROMs:
  - in supine position:
    - raise the leg above the body keeping the knee in extension – flexion
    - raise the leg above the body and then flex the knee and bring it towards the chest – flexion
    - Hold the iliac crest as the patient goes through the movement and feel when the pelvis takes over from the hip joint. This will enable an accurate measurement of range.

    - swing the leg across the body – adduction
    - swing the leg outwards – abduction
    - place the side of the patient's foot on the opposite knee and move the flexed knee towards the side of the examination couch – external rotation
    - place the side of the patient's foot on the side of the examination couch with the knee flexed and let the patient's leg fall inwards – internal rotation
- in prone or standing position:
    - ask the patient to swing the straightened leg behind the body – hyperextension

11.17.6.2 Knees

The articulation between the femur, patella, and tibia. The preferred position for knee examination is patient positioned supine on a couch.

- Inspect the knee in flexion and extension.
- Inspect for swelling, contour, and symmetry.
- Inspect the popliteal region for swelling with the knee in extension.
- Inspect the patella, particularly as the knee is flexed. Ensure that the patella tracks in a straight line and the quadriceps femoris tendon is not pulling it laterally because of the muscle being lax.
- During walking, observe for any locking of the knee or giving way – ligament injuries, loose bodies within the joint, meniscal tears.
- Palpate the suprapatella pouch, and bursae of the knee – suprapatella, prepatella, infrapatella, and semimembranous.
- Palpate the medial and lateral collateral ligaments for any pain and the cruciate ligaments.

- Palpate the patella, holding at the apex of the patella, ensure that it moves freely.
- Palpate the head of fibula and tibial tuberosity for any pain or tenderness.
- Palpate the medial and lateral joint surfaces.
- If swelling is present to the knee, test for an effusion – 'bulge sign'. Milk up the medial side of the swelling so that it disappears behind the patella, lightly tap the lateral side and the bulge will reappear. A positive bulge sign may be absent in large effusions.
- Observe the patient going through the ROMs:
    - bend the knee – flexion
    - straighten the knee – extension
    - in supine position; place your hand under the patient's knee and ask him to press down against your hand – hyperextension; if a patient has hyperextended knees, you will not be able to place your hand between the patient's knee and the examination couch
- If ligament injury is suspected, ligament instability or drawer tests should be performed; these tests are beyond the scope of this chapter; refer to texts that address sports injury.

11.17.6.3 Ankles

The articulation between the tibia, fibula, and talus.

The subtalar joint – the articulation between the calcaneum and the talus.

- Inspect the ankle during weight bearing and non-weight bearing.
- Inspect the Achilles tendon for ulcers or necrosis – damage to the Achilles tendon can result in a *foot drop*; thus the patient's foot should be inspected for plantar flexion and adduction at rest.

- Inspect the condition of the medial and lateral malleoli.
- Inspect the condition of the calcaneum.
- Inspect the ankle for swelling and contour – particularly over the anterior aspect of the ankle where swelling is more visible.
- Palpate the ankle for oedema, pain, or tenderness.
- Palpate the Achilles tendon for any pain – to test if the Achilles is intact, have the patient either kneeling or with legs hanging over the edge of an examination couch. Apply pressure just below the fullest part of the calf, if the Achilles tendon is intact the foot will plantarflex. If it does plantarflex but with pain it is the gastrocnemius muscle that is causing the problem rather than the Achilles tendon. If the Achilles tendon is ruptured, the foot will not plantarflex.
- Palpate the calcaneum for any pain.
- If spinal cord compression is suspected assess for ankle clonus.
- Observe the patient as he goes through the ROMs:
  - point the foot downwards – plantar flexion
  - point the foot upwards – dorsiflexion
  - rotate the foot laterally – abduction
  - rotate the foot medially – adduction
  - point the medial side of the foot towards the floor – eversion
  - point the lateral side of the foot towards the floor – inversion

11.17.6.4 Toes

The tarsometatarsal joint – the articulation between the distal portions of the talus and the metatarsal bones.

The metatarsalphalangeal joints – the articulation between the metatarsal bone and the proximal phalanx.

The interphalangeal joint – the articulation between the distal and proximal phalanx bones.

- Inspect each toe for calluses, corns, hammer toes and general condition of the skin.
- Inspect the hallux for evidence of valgus deformities (bunions).
- On weight bearing, inspect for the presence of an arch.
- Inspect the condition of the plantar aspect of the foot.
- Palpate each of the toes for pain or tenderness.
- Palpate for any pain on the plantar, lateral, and medial aspects of the foot.
- Provide passive movement to each of the metatarsal-phalangeal and interphalangeal joints to assess for flexion, extension, and hypertension using the index finger and thumb. Assess for any bogginess of the joints or pain elicited during movement.
- Observe the patient going through active ROMs:
  - curl up the toes – full flexion
  - straighten the toes – full extension
  - spread the toes out – abduction

11.18 Muscle Strength Tests

11.18.1 Upper Limb

- With elbows flexed, ask the patient to hold their arms above the head. You should apply pressure to the palms of their hands – deltoids.

- With arms in extension ask the patient to flex elbows; you should try and hold their arms in extension – biceps.
- With the arms flexed, ask the patient to extend them whilst you try to hold them in a flexed position – triceps.
- Ask the patient to shrug shoulders against resistance from you – trapezius. (This test will also assess the motor function of cranial nerve XI.)
- Ask the patient to maintain wrist flexion whilst you try to extend the wrist – wrist flexors.
- Ask the patient to maintain the wrist in extension as you try to flex it – wrist extensors.
- Ask patient to squeeze your first 2 fingers bilaterally to assess his grip strength.
- Ask the patient to maintain a fist whilst you try to extend the fingers.
- Ask the patient to keep fingers in extension as you try to flex them into a fist.
- Ask the patient to spread fingers out whilst you try to push them together.
- Ask the patient to put fingers together as you try to pull them apart.

11.18.2 Lower Limb

In supine position:

- Ask the patient to raise their extended leg whilst you try to hold it down – gluteals.
- Ask the patient to push their extended knees outwards against your hands – gluteals and tensor fascia lata.
- Ask the patient to push their extended knees inwards against your hands – gluteals and adductors.

- Ask the patient to extend their knee as you try to flex it – quadriceps.
- Ask the patient to flex their knee you try to extend it – hamstrings.
- Ask the patient to dorsiflex their foot against your hand – tibialis anterior and extensors.
- Ask the patient to plantarflex their foot against your hand – tibialis posterior, flexors, gastrocnemius, and soleus.
- Ask the patient to push the side of his foot against your hands.
- In sitting position (with legs hanging):
- Ask the patient to cross his legs alternately – hamstrings, gluteals, hip abductors, and hip adductors.

11.19 Terms of Location

Anterior	The front of the body.
Posterior	The back of the body.
Medial	Towards the midline of the body.
Lateral	Away from the midline of the body.
Inferior	Below, or in the direction of the bottom of the body.
Superior	Above, or in the direction of the top of the body.
Proximal	Towards the midpoint of the body, or another structure.
Distal	Away from the midpoint of the body, or another structure.
Dorsal	On, or in the direction of the back of the hand, or top of the foot.
Plantar	On, or in the direction of the sole of the foot.
Palmar	On, or in the direction of the palm of the hand.

11.20 Terms Used to Describe ROM

Flexion	To make the inner angle of the joint smaller.
Extension	To make the inner angle of the joint larger.
Abduction	To move away from the midline of the body.
Adduction	To move towards the midline of the body.
Lateral bending	Side bending.
Internal rotation	Rotating around a long axis, inwardly.
External rotation	Rotating around a long axis, outwardly.
Circumduction	Circular movement.
Dorsiflexion	To bend the ankle with the foot moving upwards.
Plantar flexion	To bend the ankle with the foot moving downwards.
Eversion	Turning the sole of the foot out.
Inversion	Turning the sole of the foot inwards.
Pronation	To rotate the forearm with the palm turning inwards.
Supination	To rotate the forearm with the palm turning outwards.
Elevation	Draw up.
Depression	Draw down.
Protraction	Draw forwards.
Retraction	Draw backwards.
Radial deviation	With palm facing down, hand moves towards from the body.
Ulnar deviation	With palm facing down, hand moves away the body.

11.21 Reference Grid for Examination

Joint	Position	Flexion	Hyperflexion	Extension	Hyperextension	Internal rotation	External rotation	Lateral rotation	Adduction	Abduction	Supination	Pronation	Dorsiflexion	Plantarflexion	Eversion	Inversion	Lateral bending	Circumduction	Radial deviation	Ulna deviation	Opposition	Depression	Elevation	Protraction	Retraction
Jaw	Sitting																								
Neck	Sitting																								
Shoulder	Standing																								
Elbow	Sitting																								
Wrist	Sitting																								
Fingers	Sitting																								
Hips	Supine																								
	Prone/ standing																								
Knees	Supine																								
Ankles	Supine																								
Toes	Supine																								
Spine (thoracic and lumbar)	Standing																								

References

Ball, J., Dains, J., Flynn, J. et al. (2014a). *Seidel's Guide to Physical Examination*, 8e. St. Louis: Mosby.

Ball, J., Dains, J., Flynn, J. et al. (2014b). *Student Laboratory Manual to Accompany Seidel's Guide to Physical Examination*, 8e. St. Louis: Mosby.

Barkauskas, V., Baumann, L., and Darling-Fisher, C. (2002). *Health and Physical Assessment*, 3e. London: Mosby.

Bickley, L. and Szilagyi, P. (2007). *Bates' Guide to Physical Examination and History Taking*, 9e. Philadelphia: Lippincott.

Bickley, L. and Szilagyi, P. (2013). *Bates' Guide to Physical Examination and History Taking*, 11e. New York: Wolters Kluwer/Lippincott Williams & Wilkins.

Bone and Joint Initiative (2014) The Burden of Musculoskeletal Diseases in the United States. http://www.boneandjointburden.org/2014-report (accessed 27 January 2018).

Dains, J., Baumann, L., and Scheibel, P. (2012). *Advanced Health Assessment and Clinical Diagnosis in Primary Care*, 4e. St. Louis: Elsevier.

Dains, J., Baumann, L., and Scheibel, P. (2015). *Advanced Health Assessment and Clinical Diagnosis in Primary Care*, 5e. St. Louis: Mosby.

Doherty, M., Dacre, J., Dieppe, P., and Snaith, M. (1992). The 'GALS' locomotor screen. *Annals of the Rheumatic Diseases* 51 (10): 1165–1169.

Epstein, O., Perkin, G., de Bono, D., and Cookson, J. (2008). *Clinical Examination*, 4e. London: Mosby.

EU Report v5.0 (2010) Musculoskeletal Health in Europe. http://www.eumusc.net/myUploadData/files/Musculoskeletal%20Health%20in%20Europe%20Report%20v5.pdf (accessed 27 January 2018).

Japp, A. and Robertson, C. (2013). *Macleod's Clinical Diagnosis*. Edinburgh: Churchill Livingstone, Elsevier.

Jarvis, C. (2008). *Physical Examination and Health Assessment*, 5e. St. Louis: Saunders.

Jarvis, C. (2015). *Physical Examination and Health Assessment*, 7e. Edinburgh: Elsevier.

Martini, F., Nath, J., and Bartholomew, E. (2012). *The Musculoskeletal System in Fundamentals of Anatomy & Physiology*, 9e. San Francisco, CA: Pearson Benjamin Cummings.

MSK (2015) Musculoskeletal Health in the Workplace: a Toolkit for Employers. https://wellbeing.bitc.org.uk/sites/default/files/business_in_the_community_musculoskeletal_toolkit.pdf (accessed 28 August 2018).

Seidel, H., Ball, J., Dains, J., and Benedict, G. (2006). *Mosby's Physical Examination Handbook*. St. Louis: Mosby.

Seidel, H., Ball, J., Dains, J., and Benedict, G. (2010). *Mosby's Physical Examination Handbook*, 7e. St. Louis: Mosby-Year Book.

Swartz, M. (2006). *Physical Diagnosis, History and Examination*, 5e. London: W. B. Saunders.

Swartz, M. (2014). *Physical Diagnosis: History and Examination*, With Student Consult Online Access, 7e. London: Elsevier.

Talley, N. and O'Connor, S. (2006). *Clinical Examination: A Systematic Guide to Physical Diagnosis*, 5e. London: Churchill Livingstone.

Talley, N. and O'Connor, S. (2014). *Clinical Examination: A Systematic Guide to Physical Diagnosis*, 7e. London: Churchill Livingstone, Elsevier.

Tallia, A. and Scherger, J. (2013). *Swanson's Family Practice Review*, 6e. St. Louis: Mosby.

Thomas, J. and Monaghan, T. (2007). *Oxford Handbook of Clinical Examination and Practical Skills*. Oxford: Oxford University Press.

Walsh, M. (2006). *Nurse Practitioners Clinical Skills and Professional Issues*, 2e. Edinburgh: Elsevier.

12

Presenting Cases and Communication

Carol Lynn Cox[1,2]
[1] *School of Health Sciences, City, University of London, London, UK*
[2] *Health and Hope Clinics, Pensacola, FL, USA*

12.1 Presentations to Healthcare Professionals and Patients

12.1.1 Introduction

Practitioners working within a healthcare system must be able to communicate effectively to other healthcare practitioners for the sake of their patients (Collins-Bride and Saxe 2013; Cox 2010, Cox and Hill 2010; Lack 2012; Rhoads and Paterson 2013). Being an advocate for your patients is one of the most important roles you portray within your practice discipline (Ball et al. 2014a, b; Bickley and Szilagyi 2013; Cox and Hill 2010; Dains et al. 2012, 2015; Japp and Robertson 2013; Jarvis 2015; Seidel et al. 2010; Swartz 2014; Talley and O'Connor 2014). The more practice you get in speaking, the better you will become and the more confident you will appear in front of other healthcare professionals and patients. Confidence displayed by you and an

Pocket Guide to Physical Assessment, First Edition. Edited by Carol Lynn Cox.

ability to speak lucidly are important aspects of therapy. Their value to the patient is enormous.

Practise talking to yourself in a mirror, avoiding any breaks or interpolating the word 'er', 'uh', or 'um'. Open a textbook, find a subject, and give a little talk on it to yourself. Even if you do not know anything about the subject, you will be able to make up a few coherent sentences once you have practised.

A presentation is not the time to demonstrate you have been thorough and have asked all questions. It a time to show you can intelligently assemble the essential facts.

In all presentations, give the salient positive findings and the relevant negative findings.

For example:

- In a patient with progressive dyspnoea, state if patient has ever smoked.
- In a patient with icterus, state whether the patient has been abroad, has had any recent injections or drugs, or contact with other jaundiced patients.

Three types of presentations are likely to be encountered: presentation of a case to a meeting, presentation of a new case on a ward/unit round, and a brief follow-up presentation.

12.1.2 Presentation of a Case to a Meeting

Presentation of a case to a group of healthcare practitioners in a meeting must be properly prepared, including visual aids as necessary. The principal details, shown on a PowerPoint® presentation for example, are helpful as a reminder to you, and the audience may more easily remember the details of a case if they 'see' as well as 'hear' them. An advantage of PowerPoint is the ability to print out the full presentation as a series of slides with spaces for the audience to write notes. Remember to keep narrative on the slides succinct. You can elaborate with your own narrative as you speak.

- Practise your presentation from beginning to end several times. Leave nothing to chance.
- Do not speak to the screen; speak to the audience.
- Do not stand in front of the data projector so that the screen is blocked by your shadow.
- Do not crack jokes, unless you are confident they are appropriate.
- Do not make sweeping statements.
- Do not make any statements that you cannot defend with references (medical research).
- Remember what you are advised to do in a court of law – dress up, stand up, speak up, shut up.
- Read up about the disease or problem beforehand so that you can answer any questions raised by the audience.
- Read recent leading articles, review or research publications on the subject and refer to these during your presentation.

In many clinical settings it is expected that you present an apposite, original article. Be prepared to evaluate and criticise the manuscript. If your seniors or colleagues cannot provide you with references, look up the subject in search engines such as CHBD, CINAHL, Medline Plus, EMBASE, Global Health, GoPubMed, HubMed, PubMed, PubPsych, British Nursing Index, Retina Medical Search, ASSIA, Cochrane Library, *Index Medicus*, or recently published textbooks (published references should be within the past five years). Always ask the librarian for advice. Laboriously repeating standard information from a textbook is often a turn-off. A recent series or research paper is more educational for you and more interesting for the audience.

A PowerPoint slide or overhead should summarise any presentation:

Mr. A. B. Age: *x* years Brief description, e.g. occupation

Complains of
(state in patient's words – for *x* period)

History of present complaint
- essential details
- other relevant information, e.g. risk factors
- relevant negative information relating to possible diagnoses
- extent to which symptoms or disease limit normal activity
- other symptoms – mention briefly

Past history
- briefly mention inactive problems
- historical information about active problems, or inactive problems relevant to present illness
- record allergies, including type of reaction to drugs

Family history
- brief information about parents, otherwise detail only if relevant
  (Present a genogram for the audience to review.)

Social history
- brief unless relevant
- give family social background
- occupation and previous occupations
- any other special problems
- tobacco or ethanol abuse, past or present

Treatment
- note all drugs with doses

Chief complaint
- note in the patient's words what the patient indicates the problem is

On examination

General description

- introductory descriptive sentence, e.g. well, obese man (indicate body mass index)
- review of systems as indicated from the patient's perspective (e.g. no complaint of skin problems or hair loss)
- clinical signs relevant to disease
- relevant negative findings

  Remember these findings should be descriptive data rather than your interpretation.

Problem list
Differential diagnoses
(Put in order of likelihood.)

Investigations

- relevant positive findings
- relevant negative findings
- tables or graphs for repetitive data
- scan an electrocardiogram or temperature chart for the PowerPoint presentation or photocopy an electrocardiogram or temperature chart for distribution to the audience

Progress report
Plan
Subjects which often are discussed after your presentation are:

- other differential diagnoses
- other features of presumed diagnosis that might have been present or require investigation
- pathophysiological mechanisms
- mechanisms of action of drugs and possible side effects.

12.1.3 Presentation of a New Case on a Ward/Unit Round

- Good written notes are of great assistance. Do not read your notes word for word – use your notes as a reference.
- Highlight, underline, or asterisk key features you wish to refer to or write up a separate notecard for reference.
- Talk formally and avoid speaking too quickly or too slowly. Speak to the whole assembled group rather than a tête-à-tête with the doctor/consultant.
- Stand upright and look presentable – it helps to make you appear confident.
- If you are interrupted by a discussion, note where you are and be ready to resume, repeating the last sentence before proceeding.

12.1.3.1 History

The format will be similar to that on PowerPoint or an overhead, with emphasis on positive findings and relevant negative information. A full description of the initial main symptom is usually required.

12.1.3.2 Examination

Once your history is complete the doctor/consultant may ask for the relevant clinical signs only. Still add relevant negative signs you think are important.

12.1.3.3 Summary

Be prepared to give a problem list and differential diagnoses.

If you are presenting the patient at the bedside, ensure the patient is comfortable. If the patient wishes to make an additional point or clarification, it is best to welcome this. If it is relevant it can be helpful. If irrelevant, politely say to the patient you will come back to them in a moment, after you have presented the findings. Do not appear to disagree with the patient in the patient's presence.

12.1.4 Brief Follow-Up Presentation

Give a brief, orienting introduction to provide a framework on which other information can be placed. For example:

> A *xx*-year-old man who was admitted *xx* days ago.
> Long-standing problems include *xxxxx* (list briefly).
> Presented with *xx* symptoms for *x* period.
> On examination had *xx* signs.
> Initial diagnosis of *xx* was confirmed/supported by/not supported by *xx* investigations.
> He was treated by *xx*.
> Since then *xx* progress:
>
> - symptoms
> - examination
>   Start with general description and temperature chart and, if relevant, investigations.
>
> If there are multiple active problems, describe each separately, e.g.
>
> - first in regard to the *xxxx*
> - second in regard to the *xxxx*
>
> The outstanding problems are *xxxx*.
> The plan is *xxxx*.

12.1.5 Aides-Mémoire

These are basic lists that provide brief reminders when presenting patients and diseases. Organising your thoughts along structured lines is helpful.

12.1.5.1 History

- principal symptom(s)
- history of present illness
- note chronology
- present situation
- functional enquiry
- past history
- family history
- personal and social history

12.1.5.2 Pain or Other Symptoms

- site
- radiation
- character
- severity
- onset/duration
- frequency/periodicity or constant
- precipitating factors
- relieving factors
- associated symptoms
- getting worse or better

12.1.5.3 Lumps

12.1.5.3.1 Inspection

- site
- size
- shape
- surface
- surroundings

12.1.5.3.2 Palpation

- soft/solid consistency
- surroundings – fixed/mobile
- tender
- pulsatility
- transmission of illumination

12.1.5.3.3 Local Lymph Nodes

Delineate nodes in the occipital region, cervical region, neck, axillary, or groin, for example.

12.1.5.4 About the Disease

- incidence
- geographical area
- gender/age
- aetiology
- pathology
  - macroscopic
  - microscopic
- pathophysiology
- symptoms
- signs
- therapy
- prognosis

12.1.5.5 Causes of Disease

- genetic
- infective
  - virus
  - bacterial
  - fungal
  - parasitic
- neoplastic
  - cancer
    - primary
    - secondary
  - lymphoma
- vascular
  - atheroma
  - hypertension
  - other, e.g. arteritis

- infiltrative
    - fibrosis
    - amyloid
    - granuloma
- autoimmune
- endocrine
- degenerative
- environmental
    - trauma
    - iatrogenic – drug side effects
    - poisoning
- malnutrition
    - general
    - specific, e.g. vitamin deficiency
    - perinatal with effects on subsequent development

12.1.6 Diagnostic Labels

- aetiology, e.g. tuberculosis, genetic
  ↓
- pathology, e.g. sarcoid, amyloid
  ↓
- disordered function, e.g. hypertension, diabetes
  ↓
- symptoms or signs, e.g. jaundice, erythema nodosum

12.2 People – Including Patients

A significant number of disasters, a great deal of irritation, and a lot of unpleasantness could be avoided in the general practice surgery, outpatient clinics, primary care facilities, and hospitals by proper communication. You must remember that you are part of a multidisciplinary team, all of whom significantly help the patient. You must be able to communicate properly with the medical staff, nursing staff, physiotherapists, occupational therapists, administrators, ancillary staff, and, above all, the patients.

Remember these points.

- Time – when you talk to anyone, try not to appear in a rush or they will lose concentration and not listen. A little time taken to talk to somebody properly will help enormously. One minute spent sitting down can seem like five minutes to the patient; five minutes standing up can seem like one minute.
- Silence – in normal social interaction we tend to avoid silences. In a conversation, as soon as one person stops talking (or even before) the other person jumps in to say their bit. When interviewing patients, it is often useful, if you wish to encourage the patient to talk further, to remain silent a moment longer than would be natural. An encouraging nod of the head or an echoing of the patient's last word or two (reflection) may also encourage the patient to talk further.
- Listen – active listening is not easy but essential for good communication. Many people stop talking but not all appear to be listening. Sitting down with the patient is advantageous, both in helping you to concentrate and in transmitting to the patient that you are willing to listen.
- Smile and use facilitative body language – grumpiness or irritation is the best way to stop a patient talking. A smile and display of interest will often encourage a patient to tell you problems they would not normally do. This behaviour helps everybody to relax.
- Reassurance – if you appear confident and relaxed this helps others to feel the same. Being calm without excessive body movements can help. Note how a

good advanced nurse practitioner has a reassuring word for patients and allows others in the team to feel they are (or are capable of) working effectively.
- Advocacy – you are the patient's advocate. Advocacy is essential in order to preserve the practitioner–patient relationship.

References

Ball, J., Dains, J., Flynn, J. et al. (2014a). *Seidel's Guide to Physical Examination*, 8e. St. Louis: Mosby.

Ball, J., Dains, J., Flynn, J. et al. (2014b). *Student Laboratory Manual to Accompany Seidel's Guide to Physical Examination*, 8e. St. Louis: Mosby.

Bickley, L. and Szilagyi, P. (2013). *Bates' Guide to Physical Examination and History Taking*, 11e. New York: Wolters Kluwer/Lippincott Williams & Wilkins.

Collins-Bride, G. and Saxe, J. (2013). *Clinical Guidelines for Advanced Practice Nursing – An Interdisciplinary Approach*, 2e. Burlington, MA: Jones and Bartlett Learning.

Cox, C. (2010). *Physical Assessment for Nurses*, 2e. Oxford: Wiley Blackwell.

Cox, C. and Hill, M. (2010). *Professional Issues in Primary Care Nursing*. Oxford: Wiley Blackwell.

Dains, J., Baumann, L., and Scheibel, P. (2012). *Advanced Health Assessment and Clinical Diagnosis in Primary Care*, 4e. St. Louis: Elsevier.

Dains, J., Baumann, L., and Scheibel, P. (2015). *Advanced Health Assessment and Clinical Diagnosis in Primary Care*, 5e. St. Louis: Mosby.

Japp, A. and Robertson, C. (2013). *Macleod's Clinical Diagnosis*. Edinburgh: Churchill Livingstone, Elsevier.

Jarvis, C. (2015). *Physical Examination and Health Assessment*, 7e. Edinburgh: Elsevier.

Lack, V. (2012). Consultation skills. In: *Advanced Practice in Healthcare* (ed. C. Cox, M. Hill and V. Lack), 39–56. London: Routledge.

Rhoads, J. and Paterson, S. (2013). *Advanced Health Assessment and Diagnostic Reasoning*, 2e. Burlington: Jones and Bartlett.

Seidel, H., Ball, J., Dains, J., and Benedict, G. (2010). *Mosby's Physical Examination Handbook*, 7e. St. Louis: Mosby-Year Book.

Swartz, M. (2014). *Physical Diagnosis: History and Examination*, with Student Consult Online Access, 7e. London: Elsevier.

Talley, N. and O'Connor, S. (2014). *Clinical Examination: A Systematic Guide to Physical Diagnosis*, 7e. London: Churchill Livingstone, Elsevier.

Appendix A

Jaeger Reading Chart

Jaeger types assess visual acuity for close tasks. They provide the easiest quick method of assessment. The patient should wear the spectacles normally required for reading. Ask the patient to read the smallest type she can; if read with few mistakes, ask her to read the next size down. Record the size of type that can be read with each eye separately.

Hope, they say, deserts us at no period of our existence. From First to last, and in the face of smarting disillusions we continue to expect good fortune, better health, and better conduct; and that so confidently, that we judge it needless to deserve them. I think it improbable that I shall ever write like Shakespeare, conduct an army like Hannibal, or distinguish

Here we recognise the thoughts of our boyhood; and our boyhood ceased – well, when? – not, I think, at twenty: nor, perhaps, altogether at twenty-five: nor yet at thirty: and possibly to be quite frank, we are still in the thick of that arcadian period. For as the race of man, after centuries of civilisation, still keeps

I have always suspected public taste to be a mongrel product, out of affectation by dogmatism; and felt sure, if you could only find an honest man of no special literary

Pocket Guide to Physical Assessment, First Edition. Edited by Carol Lynn Cox.

bent, he would tell you he thought much of Shakespeare bombastic and most absurd, and all of him written in very

If you look back on your own education, I am sure it will not be the full, vivid, instructive hours of truancy that you regret: and you would rather cancel some lacklustre period between sleep and waking in the class. For my own part, I have attended

There is a sort of dead-alive, hackneyed people about, who are scarcely conscious of living except in the exercise of some conventional occupation.

Books are good enough in their own way, but they are a mighty bloodless substitute for life. It seems a pity to sit, like the Lady of Shalott, peering into a mirror,

The other day, a ragged, barefoot boy ran down the street after a marble, with so jolly an air that he set every one he passed

A happy man or woman is a better thing to find than a

"How now, young fellow, what dost thou

"Truly, sir, I

Reference

Hatton, C. and Blackwood, R. (2003). *Lecture Notes on Clinical Skills*, 4e. Oxford: Blackwell Sciences LTD.

Appendix B

Visual Acuity 3 Meter/21 Foot Chart

The 3m Snellen chart should be held 3 m (21 feet) from the patient, with good lighting, with each of the patient's eyes covered in turn. Use the patient's usual spectacles/glasses for this distance. If the patient cannot read 6/6 (United Kingdom) or 20/20 (North America) (e.g. 6/12 = UK or 20/12 = NA is best vision in one eye), repeat without spectacles/glasses and with a 'pinhole' that largely nullifies refractive errors. Note for each eye the best acuity obtained and the method used, e.g. L 6/9 R 6/6 with spectacles or L 20/7 R 20/7 with glasses.

Reference

Hatton, C. and Blackwood, R. (2003). *Lecture Notes on Clinical Skills*, 4e. Oxford: Blackwell Sciences LTD.

Pocket Guide to Physical Assessment, First Edition. Edited by Carol Lynn Cox.

Appendix C

Hodkinson Ten-Point Mental Test Score

A simple test of impaired cognitive function.

1. Age	Must be correct
2. Time	Without looking at clock or watch, and correct to nearest hour
3. 42 West Street	Give this (or similar) address twice, ask patient to repeat immediately (to check it has registered), and test recall at end of procedure
4. Recognise two people	Point at nurse and other, ask: 'Who is that person? What does she/he do?'
5. Year	Exact, except in January when previous year is accepted
6. Name of place	May ask type of place or area of town
7. Date of birth	Exact
8. Start of World War I	Exact year
9. Name of present monarch	
10. Count from 20 to 1	Backwards, may prompt with 20/19/18, no other prompts; patient may hesitate and self-correct but no other errors (tests concentration)

Check recall of address (question 3 above)

Total score out of 10

Communication problems (e.g. *deafness, dysphasia*) or abnormal mood (e.g. *depression*) may affect the mental test score, and should be noted. (Source: After Qureshi and Hodkinson (1974).)

Reference

Qureshi, K. and Hodkinson, H. (1974). Evaluation of a ten-question mental test in the institutional elderly. *Age and Ageing* 3: 152.

Appendix D

Barthel Index of Activities of Daily Living

An assessment of disabilities affecting key functions that influence a person's mobility, self-care, and independence.

Bowels

0 = incontinent (or needs to be given enema)
1 = occasional accident (once per week or less)
2 = continent (for preceding week)

Bladder

0 = incontinent or catheterised and unable to manage alone
1 = occasional accident (once per day or less)
2 = continent (for preceding week)

Feeding

0 = unable
1 = needs help cutting, spreading butter, etc.
2 = independent

Pocket Guide to Physical Assessment, First Edition. Edited by Carol Lynn Cox.

Grooming

0 = needs help with personal care

1 = independent face/hair/teeth/shaving (implements provided)

Dressing

0 = dependent

1 = needs help but can do about half unaided

2 = independent (including buttons, zips, laces, etc.)

Transfer bed to chair and back

0 = unable, no sitting balance

1 = major help (one strong/skilled or two people), can sit up

2 = minor help from one person (physical or verbal)

3 = independent

Toilet use

0 = dependent

1 = needs some help, but can do something alone

2 = independent (on and off, dressing, wiping)

Mobility around house or ward, indoors

0 = immobile

1 = wheelchair independent, including corners

2 = walks with help of one person (physical, verbal, supervision)

3 = independent (but may use any aid, e.g. stick)

Stairs

0 = unable

1 = needs help (physical, verbal, carrying aid)

2 = independent

Bathing

0 = dependent
1 = independent (in and out of bath or shower)

Total score out of 20

Guidelines for the Barthel Index of Activities of Daily Living (ADL)

1. The index should be used as a record of what a patient does, not what a patient *can* do.
2. The main aim is to establish the degree of independence from any help, physical or verbal, however minor and for whatever reason.
3. The need for supervision renders the patient not independent.
4. A patient's performance should be established using the best available evidence. The patient, friends/relatives and nurses are the usual sources, but direct observation and common sense are also important. Direct testing is not necessary.
5. Usually the patient's performance over the preceding 24–48 hours is important, but occasionally longer periods will be relevant.
6. Middle categories imply that the patient supplies over 50% of the effort.
7. The use of aids to be independent is allowed.

(Source: After Collin et al. (1988).)

Reference

After Collin, C., Wade, D.T., Davies, S., and Horne, V. (1988). The Barthel ADL index: a reliability study. *International Disability Studies* 10: 61–63.

Appendix E

Mini-Mental State Examination (MMSE)

The purpose of the Mini-Mental State Examination (MMSE) is to determine the mental status of a patient. It should be incorporated into mental health and neurological assessments as well as being an essential component of examinations in which dementia is suspected in the older adult. The MMSE may be viewed as the psychological equivalent of a physical examination. Through utilisation of the MMSE it is possible to evaluate both quantitatively and qualitatively a range of mental functions and behaviours at specific points in time (House 2016). The MMSE is beneficial in obtaining important information related to cognitive functioning that is used in formulating a diagnosis and discerning a disorder's progression and response to treatment. In addition to the scores obtained from the various tests shown here, observations of the patient during the interview should become part of the MMSE, which begins when the healthcare professional initially meets the patient. Information gathered includes the patient's behaviours, thinking, and mood. The healthcare professional's informal and formal observations should be integrated from the assessment tools shown in this appendix. The sum total of these tools provide substantial information about the patient's attention span, memory, and organisation of thought.

Pocket Guide to Physical Assessment, First Edition. Edited by Carol Lynn Cox.

The MMSEs shown here include information about appearance, motor activity, speech, affect, thought content, thought process, perception, intellect, and insight.

Major Elements of the Mental Status Examination

Appearance: Age, sex, race, body build, posture, eye contact, dress, grooming, manner, attentiveness to examiner, distinguishing features, prominent physical abnormalities, emotional facial expression, alertness.

Motor: Retardation, agitation, abnormal movements, gait, catatonia.

Speech: Rate, rhythm, volume, amount, articulation, spontaneity.

Affect: Stability, range, appropriateness, intensity, affect, mood.

Thought content: Suicidal ideation, death wishes, homicidal ideation, depressive cognitions, obsessions, ruminations, phobias, ideas of reference, paranoid ideation, magical ideation, delusions, overvalued ideas.

Thought process: Associations, coherence, logic, stream, clang associations, perseveration, neologism, blocking, attention.

Perception: Hallucinations, illusions, depersonalization, derealisation, déjà vu, jamais vu.

Intellect: Global impression: average, above average, below average.

Insight: Awareness of illness.

Source: Adapted from Zimmerman (1994, pp. 121–122) and House (2016).

Mini-Mental State Examination

Maximum score	Patient's score	Orientation
5		What is the (year) (season) (date) (day) (month)?
5		Where are we: (state) (country) (town) (hospital) (floor)?
		Registration
3		Name three objects: take one second to say each. Then ask patient to repeat them. Give one point for each correct answer.
		Attention and calculation
5		Serials 7s from 100. One point for each correct answer. Stop after five answers. Alternatively, spell "world" backwards.
3		**Recall**
		Ask for the three objects named above. One point for each correct answer.
		Language
2		Ask patient to name a pencil and watch. (two points)
2		Repeat the following: "No ifs, ands, or buts." (two points)
3		Follow a three-stage command: "Take a paper in your right hand, fold it in half, and put it on the table." (three points)
1		Read and obey the following:
		Close your eyes (one point)

Maximum score	Patient's score	Orientation
1		Write a sentence (one point)
1		Copy a drawing of intersecting pentagons (one point)
Maximum Total = 30 (Guide: Mild >21; Moderate = 10–20; Severe < or = 9)	Actual Score =	

Source: Adapted from Folstein et al. (1975).

References

Folstein, M.F., Folstein, S.E., and McHugh, P.R. (1975). Mini-Mental State: A practical method for grading the cognitive states of patients for the clinician. *J Psychiatr Res* 12: 189–198.

House, R. (2016). The Mental Status Examination. http://www.brown.edu/Courses/BI_278/Other/Clerkship/Didactics/Readings/THE%20MENTAL%20STATUS%20EXAMINATION.pdf (accessed 17 August 2016).

Zimmerman, M. (1994). *Interviewing Guide for Evaluating DSM-IV Psychiatric Disorders and the Mental Status Examination, 121–122*. Philadelphia: Psychiatric Press Products.

Appendix F
Glasgow Coma Scale

The Glasgow Coma Scale (**GCS**) is a neurological scale that is considered, internationally, to be the key instrument used to determine and record the conscious state of a patient.

Glasgow Coma Scale

Category	Score
Eyes open (E)	
Spontaneously 4	
To speech 3	
To pain 2	
None 1	
Best motor response (M)	
Obeys command 5	
Localises pain 4	
Flexion to pain 3	
Extension to pain 2	
None 1	

Pocket Guide to Physical Assessment, First Edition. Edited by Carol Lynn Cox.

Category	Score
Best verbal response (V)	
Oriented 5	
Confused 4	
Inappropriate words 3	
Incomprehensible sounds 2	
None 1	

Summed coma scale = E + M + V

Reference

Smith, S., Duell, D., and Martin, B. (2008). *Clinical Nursing Skills, Basic to Advanced Skills*, 293. London: Pearson Education LTD.

Appendix G

Warning Signs of Alzheimer's Disease

The example shown here is a good instrument for determining the executive function of a patient with potential Alzheimer's disease.

Ten Warning Signs of Alzheimer's Disease

Normal aging events	Possible Alzheimer's disease
Periodically/temporarily forgetting a person's name	Unable to remember the person discussed or seen later
Forgetting food cooking on the stove until after the meal has finished	Forgetting a meal has been prepared
Substitution of fit words because the individual is unable to remember the right word	Speaking in incomprehensible sentences
Forgetting where the person is going	Getting lost on the person's own street – unable to find their way home
Speaking on the telephone and forgetting to watch a child they are responsible for watching	Forgetting a child is present
Experiencing trouble balancing a checkbook	No longer knows what numbers mean

Pocket Guide to Physical Assessment, First Edition. Edited by Carol Lynn Cox.

Normal aging events	Possible Alzheimer's disease
Misplacing an item until retracing their steps	Putting an item in the wrong place (e.g. a wallet in the refrigerator)
Feeling the day has been depressing	Experiencing rapid mood shifts (e.g. getting angry about something inappropriately and then laughing inappropriately)
Changes in personality over time	Significant change in personality (e.g. a kind and considerate person becomes cruel and verbally abusive or inappropriate)
Getting tired of household chores but does go back and complete them later on	Does not know that household chores need to be done or caring about them

Source: Adapted from Needham (2014).

Reference

Needham, J. (2014). *Alzheimer's Disease*. Sacramento, CA: NetCE.

Appendix H

Trigger Symptoms Indicative of Dementia

Dementia is a common feature in the ageing process. When assessing a patient for dementia consider whether the patient has difficulty in any of the following areas whilst also considering how long the symptoms have been present, whether they are abrupt or gradual in onset, and whether there has been continuous or stepwise deterioration.

Trigger Symptoms of Dementia

Area of concern	Trigger symptoms
Learning/ Retaining New Information	More repetitive; trouble remembering recent conversations, events, or appointments; and more frequently misplaces items
Handling Complex Activities	Difficulty following a complex train of thought, undertaking tasks that require numerous steps (e.g. balancing a checkbook)
Ability to Reason	Unable to develop a reasonable plan to resolve problems at work or at home (e.g. what to do if the kitchen sink overflows or demonstrates an uncharacteristic disregard for social norms)

Pocket Guide to Physical Assessment, First Edition. Edited by Carol Lynn Cox.

Area of concern	Trigger symptoms
Special Abilities and Orientation	Difficulty driving, putting objects in the wrong location (e.g. putting milk from the refrigerator in the bedroom closet) or finding their way to and from familiar places. In addition, fails to arrive at the right time for appointments; has difficulty discussing current events and is untidy in dress or inappropriately dressed
Language	Difficulty in finding the correct words to express what they want to say and with following conversations (when hearing is not a problem)
Behaviour	Is passive and less responsive; is more irritable than in the past and is more suspicious (e.g. refuses having a cleaner come to clean because they might take something) and also misinterprets visual or auditory stimuli

Source: Adapted from Folstein et al. (1975) and Ferris et al. (1997).

References

Ferris, S., Mackell, J., Mohs, R. et al. (1997). A multicenter evaluation of new treatment efficacy instruments for Alzheimer's disease clinical trials: overview and general results. *Alzheimer Disease Association Disorder* 11 (supplement 1): S1–S12.

Folstein, M., Folstein, S., and McHugh, R. (1975). "Mini-Mental State": a practical method for grading the cognitive state of patients for the clinician. *Journal of Psychiatric Review* 12: 189–198.

Appendix I
The 12-Lead Electrocardiogram

I.1 General Principles

I.1.1 Introduction

The electrocardiogram (ECG) tracings arise from the electrical changes, depolarization and repolarization that accompany muscle contraction. With knowledge of the relative position of the leads to the electrodes, the ECG tracings provide direct information of the cardiac muscle and its activity.

Six **standard leads** – I, II, III, aVR, aVL, aVF – are recorded from the limb electrodes (aV = augmented voltage) and examine the heart from different directions (Figure I.1). The standard leads examine the heart in the **vertical** plane (Figure I.2).

Six **chest leads**, V leads, attached by sticky electrodes to the chest wall, are all in the **horizontal** plane (Figure I.3).

Pocket Guide to Physical Assessment, First Edition. Edited by Carol Lynn Cox.

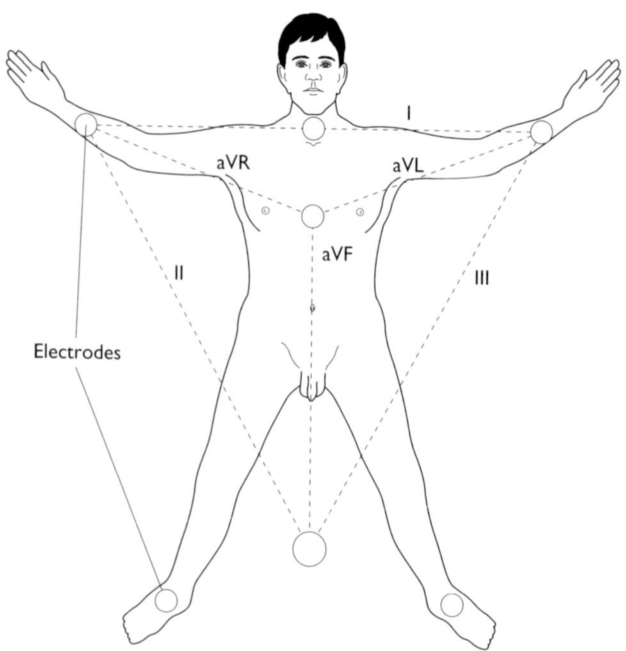

Figure I.1 The positioning of the limb electrodes and the six standard leads.

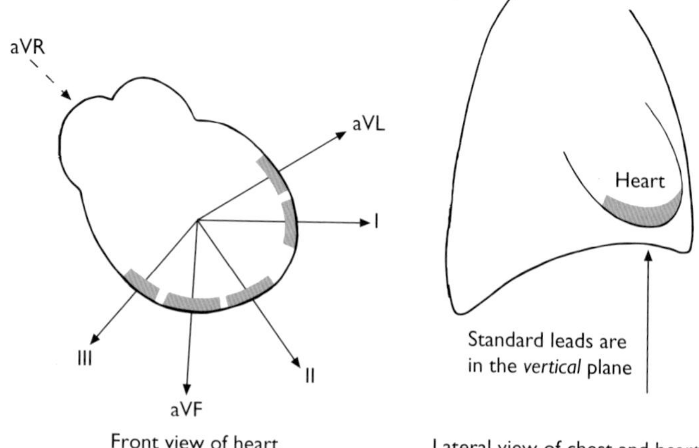

Figure I.2 Examining the vertical plane.

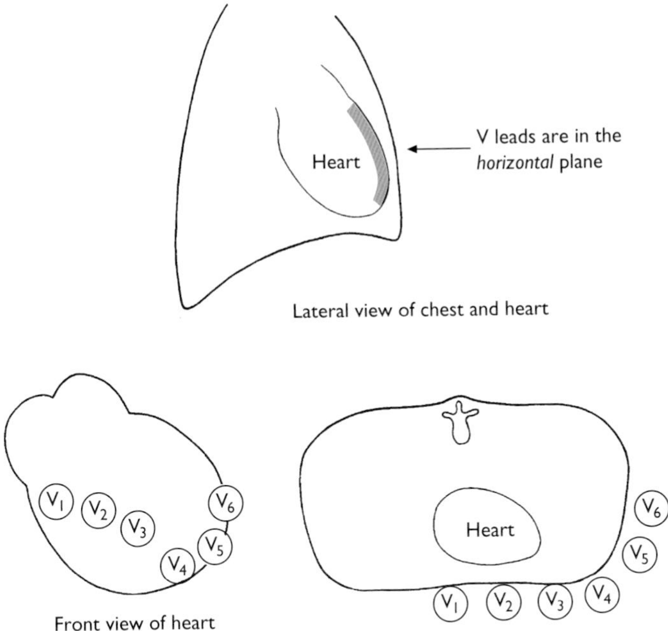

Figure I.3 Examining the horizontal plane.

Obstruction of arteries gives appropriate specific patterns of ischaemia:

- left anterior descending coronary artery – *anterior ischaemia* or *infarct* (V_{1-6})
- circumflex coronary artery – *lateral ischaemia* or *infarct* (I, aVL)
- right coronary artery – *inferior ischaemia* or *infarct* (II, III, aVF) (Figure I.4).

Every ECG tracing must first be standardised by making sure the 1 mV mark deviates the pointer 10 small squares on the paper (Figure I.5).

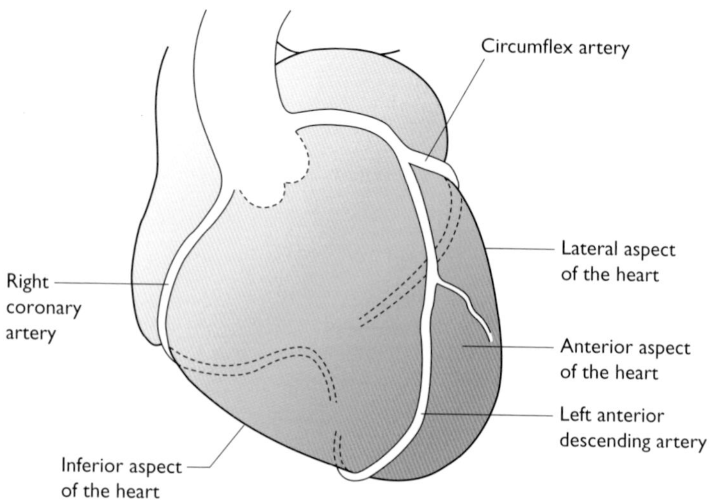

Figure I.4 Coronary arteries.

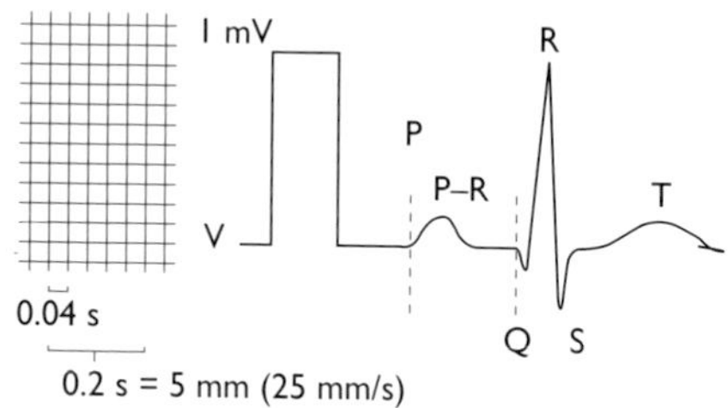

Figure I.5 Standardising the electrocardiogram (ECG) tracing. P, atrial depolarization; QRS, ventricular depolarization; T, repolarization.

I.2 Normal ECG (Figure I.6)

I.2.1 Normal ECG Variants

- T waves can be inverted in leads III, aVF, V_{1-3}.
- T waves and P waves are always inverted in aVR (if not, leads are misplaced).

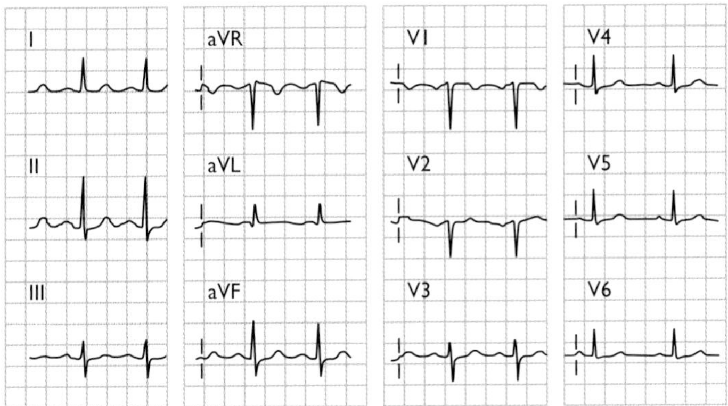

Figure I.6 A normal electrocardiogram (ECG).

- In a young athletic person:
  - ST segments may be raised, especially in leads V_{1-5}
  - right bundle branch block (RBBB) may occur
  - electrical criteria of left ventricular hypertrophy may be present
  - bradycardia < 40 beats min^{-1}
  - physiological Q waves.
- Ectopics of any type, including ventricular, are rarely of significance.
- Raised ST segments are common in Afro-Caribbean subjects.
- P mitrale is overdiagnosed:
  - P wave in V_1 is often biphasic.

I.3 Electrophysiology of Cardiac Contractions

All cardiac muscle has a tendency to depolarization, leading to excitation and contraction.

Initial electrical discharge from the sinoatrial (SA) node (under the influence of sympathetic and parasympathetic

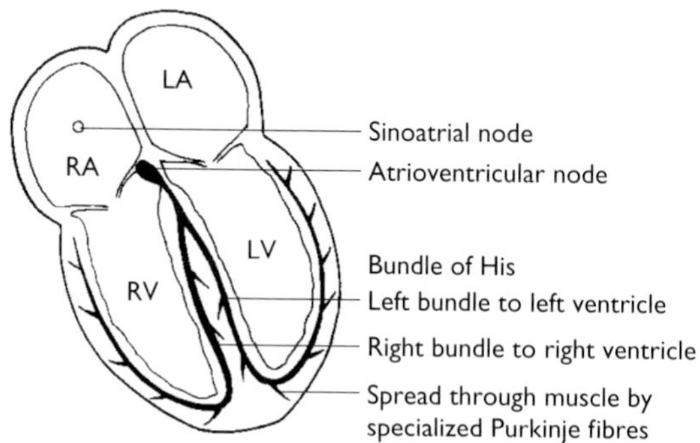

Figure I.7 Conduction system (electrical pathway).

control) spreads to the atrioventricular (AV) node and via the bundle of His to the ventricles (Figure I.7).

The deflection of the ECG tracing indicates the average direction of all muscle activity at each moment.

Depolarization spreads:

- towards lead – ECG tracing moves up the paper
- away from lead – tracing moves down paper.

I.3.1 P Wave (Figure I.8)

- depolarization spreads from SA node to AV node through the atrial muscle fibres (1 in Figure I.8)
- best seen in leads II and V_1
- usually small, as atria are small

Normal P wave <2.5 mm high, <2.5 mm wide.

I.3.2 QRS Complex (Figure I.9)

The QRS deflections have a standard nomenclature:

Q – any initial deflection downwards.

R – any deflection upwards, whether or not a preceding Q.

S – any deflection downwards after an R wave, whether or not a preceding Q.

Sinoatrial node

(1)

Normal P wave

Lead II

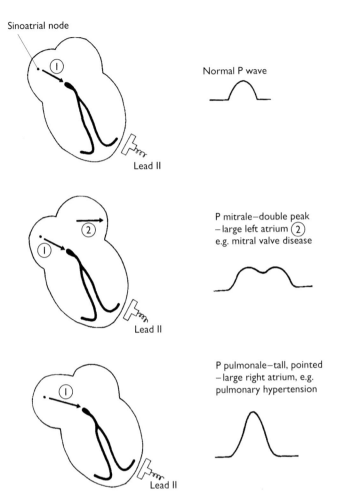

P mitrale–double peak
–large left atrium (2)
e.g. mitral valve disease

(2)

(1)

Lead II

P pulmonale–tall, pointed
–large right atrium, e.g.
pulmonary hypertension

(1)

Lead II

Figure I.8 Sinoatrial (SA) node P wave.

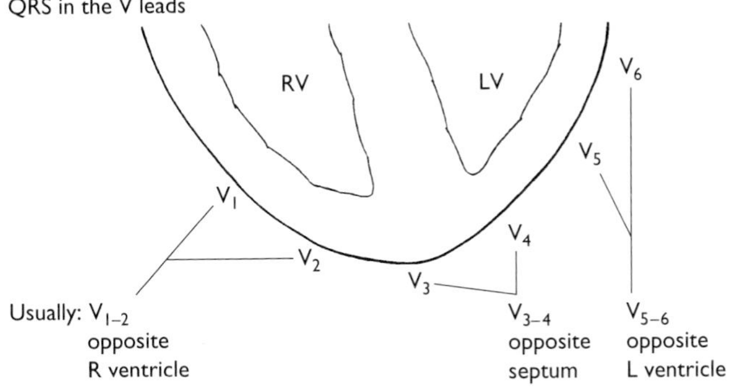

Figure I.9 QRS in the V leads.

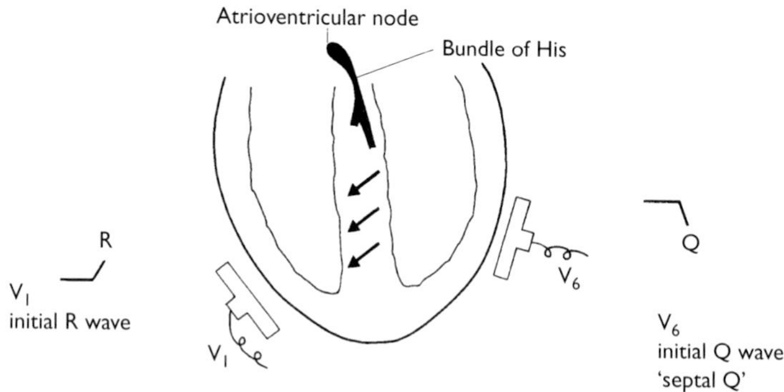

Figure I.10 Depolarization of the septum.

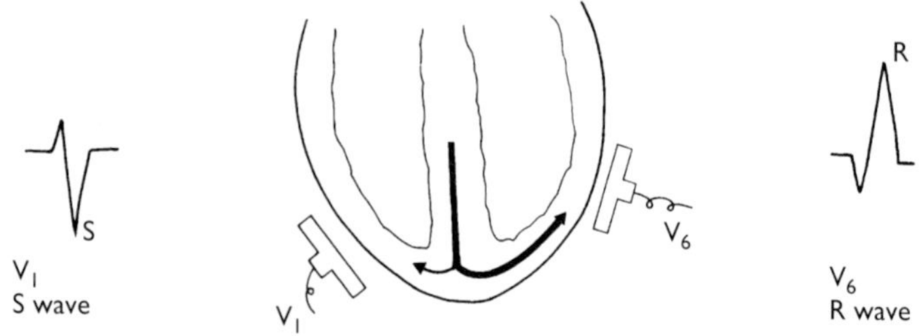

Figure I.11 Depolarization of the ventricles.

The septum depolarizes first from left to right (Figure I.10). The ventricles then depolarize from inside outwards. The large left ventricle then normally dominates (Figure I.11).

The transition point where R and S are equal is the position of the septum (Figure I.12).

V_6 S wave after R wave as depolarization spreads around ventricle away from V_6.

I.3.3 Left Ventricle Hypertrophy (LVH)

V_5 or V_6 – R wave >25 mm.

V_1 or V_2 – S wave deep.

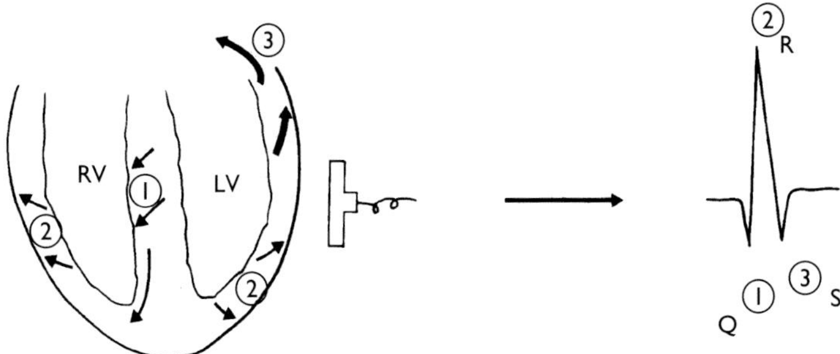

Figure I.12 The transition point.

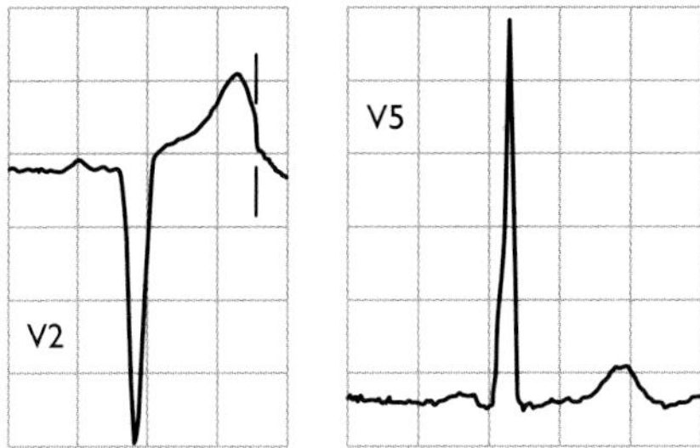

Figure I.13 Left ventricular hypertrophy.

Tallest R wave + deepest S wave >35 mm (Figure I.13).

- Voltage changes on their own are not enough – thin people with a thin ribcage can have big complexes.
- Obese people have small complexes.
- Also look for R wave in V_1
- rotation to right of transition point left axis deviation.
- T wave inversion in V_5, V_6 in the presence of left ventricle hypertrophy (LVH) is termed left ventricular 'strain pattern' and indicates marked hypertrophy (Figure I.14).

I.3.4 Right Ventricle Hypertrophy (RVH)

The left ventricle is no longer dominant.

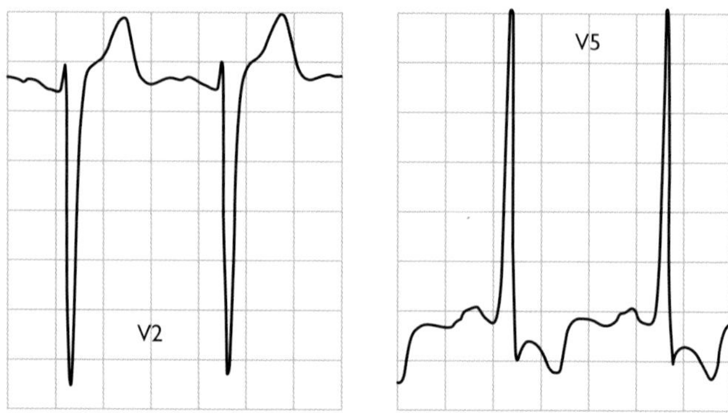

Figure I.14 Left ventricular hypertrophy strain pattern.

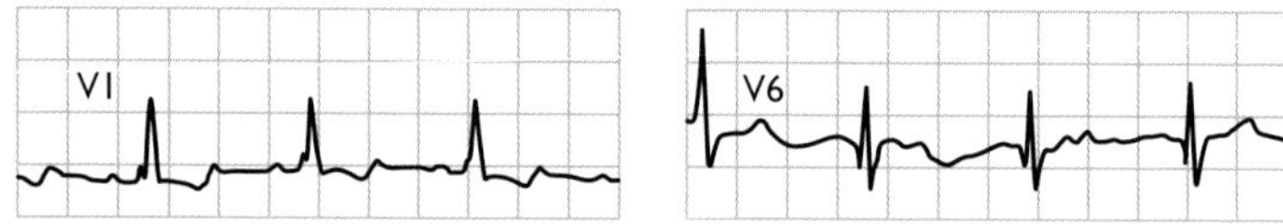

Figure I.15 Right ventricular hypertrophy.

V_1 – R wave > S wave.
V_6 – deep S wave (Figure I.15).
Also look for:

- right axis deviation
- peaked P of right atrial hypertrophy
- T wave inversion in V_2 and V_3 – right ventricular 'strain pattern'.

I.3.5 Myocardial Infarction (MI) – Full Thickness of Ventricle

Infarction is the term for dead muscle. See Table I.1 for the time sequence of ECG changes in myocardial infarction.

Table I.1 Classic time sequence of onset of electrocardiogram (ECG) changes in myocardial infarction.

Approximate time of onset after chest pain		Electrocardiogram (ECG) changes
Immediately	1. May be normal	ECG may be normal. Occasionally ST segment changes occur immediately pain develops, or even before
0–2 hours	2. 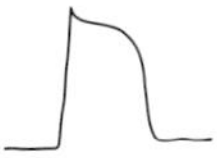	ST segments rise – occluded artery → injury pattern
3–8 hours	3. 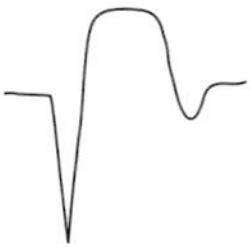	Injured tissue remains Some dies (Q waves = myocardium death) Some improves to become ischaemic only (T wave inversion) Full infarct pattern: ■ Q waves ■ raised ST segments ■ inverted T waves
8–24 hours	4. 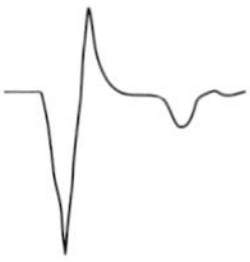	Injured tissue either dies → Q wave or improves and abnormal ST segments disappear Inverted T waves remain
After 1–2 days	5. 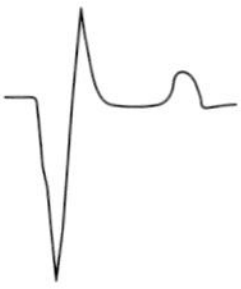	Ischaemia disappears T waves upright again Q waves usually remain, as dead tissue will not come alive again Q waves may subsequently disappear if scarred tissue contracts

I.3.6 Pathological Q Wave

- width = or > 0.04 second (one small square)
- depth > one-third height of R wave
- smaller Q waves are physiological from septum depolarization
- as ventricles depolarize from inside, an electrode in the ventricle cavity would record contraction as Q wave
- through 'dead' window, this is seen as if from inside the heart, i.e. the depolarization of the far ventricle wall away from the electrode gives a negative deflection (Figure I.16).

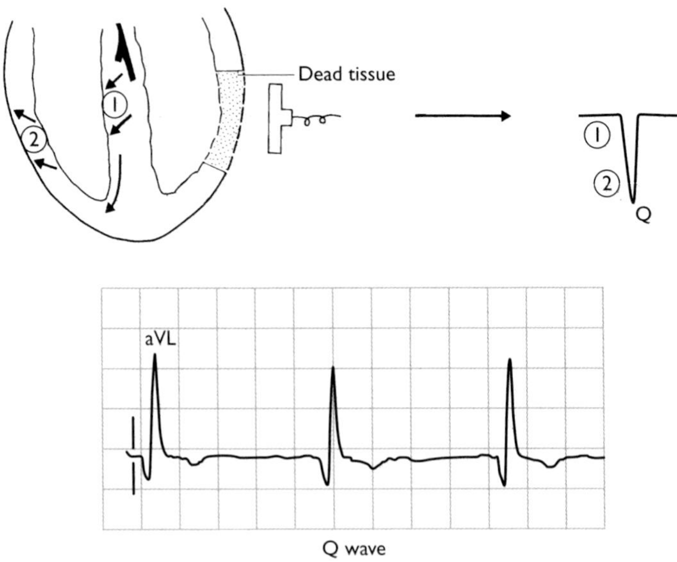

Figure I.16 Pathological Q wave.

I.3.7 Acute Myocardial Ischaemia – Raised ST Segments

I.3.7.1 Damaged but Potentially Salvageable Myocardium

- ST segment – normally within 0.5 mm of isoelectric line
- ST elevation in V_1 and V_2 may be normal – high 'take-off' of j point
- ST elevation elsewhere is normal.

I.3.7.2 Normal Baseline

Resting myocardial cell potential approximately −90 mV. In an injured cell, failing cell membrane only allows potential of perhaps −40 mV (Figure I.17).

If two electrodes record from different areas of the resting heart, one normal and one injured, a galvanometer would register −50 mV (i.e. the difference between −90 and − 40 mV). This depresses the baseline below normal over the injured area, although this cannot be recognised until after the QRS complex (Figure I.18).

Raised ST segment:

- acute ischaemic injury of ventricle
- pericarditis
- normal athletes
- normal Afro-Caribbeans.

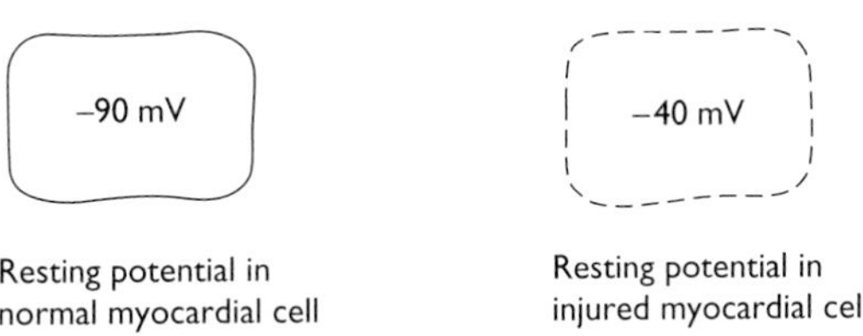

Figure I.17 Normal baseline.

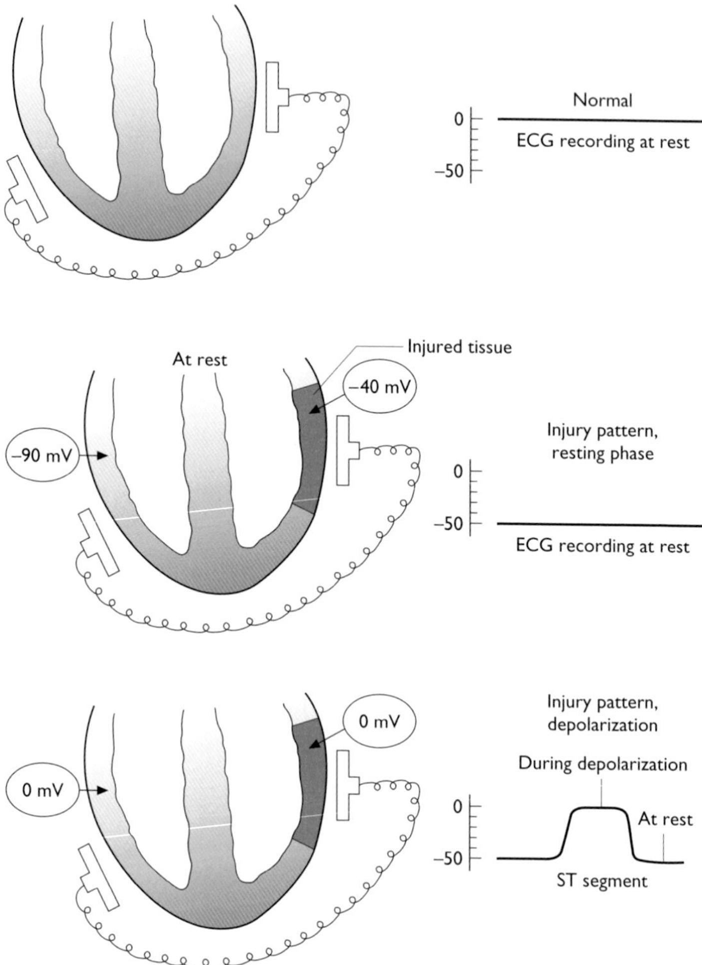

Figure I.18 Baseline changes in myocardial injury.

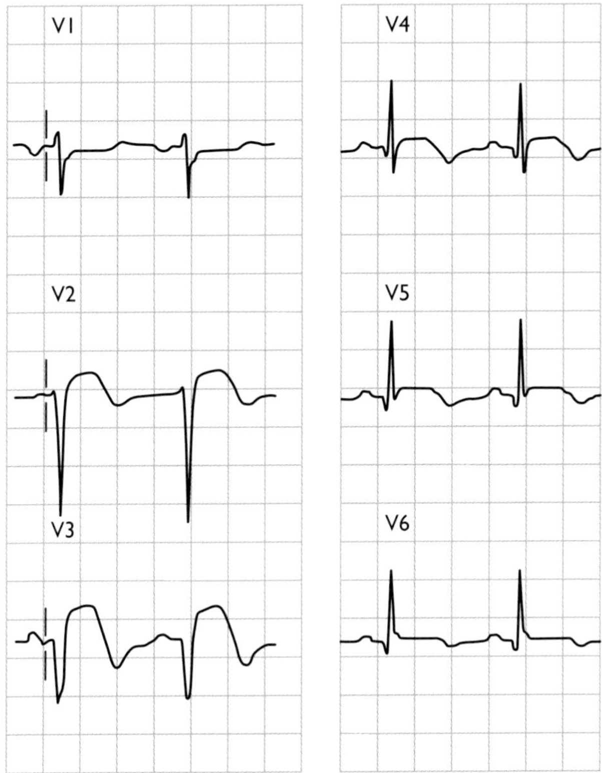

Figure I.19 Acute anterior infarct: ST ↑ V_{2-6} at three to eight hours.

I.3.8 Anterior Infarction (Figures I.19 and I.20)

- changes in leads V_{1-6}
- occlusion of left anterior descending coronary artery

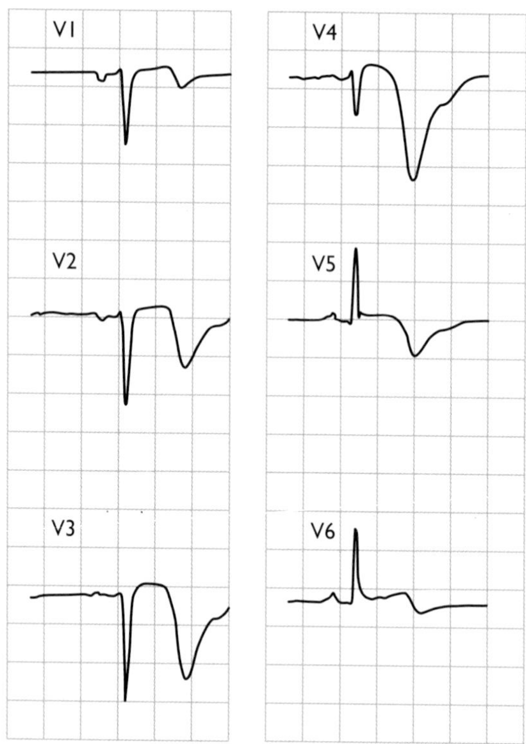

Figure I.20 Ten hours after anterior myocardial infarct.

I.3.9 Inferior Infarction (Figure I.21)

- changes in leads II, III, aVF
- occlusion of right coronary artery

I.3.10 Lateral Infarction

- changes in leads I, aVL
- occlusion of circumflex artery

I.3.11 Septal Infarction

- changes in leads V_{2-3}
- occlusion of septal branches of left anterior descending coronary artery

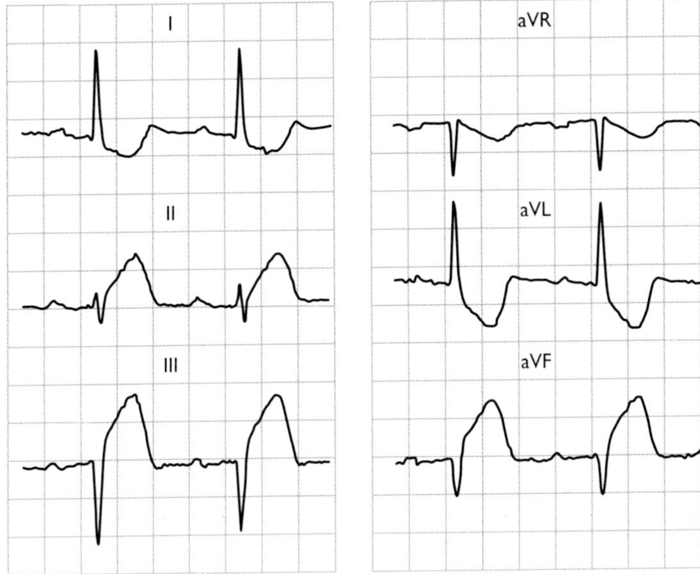

Figure I.21 Acute inferior infarct: ST · in II, III, aVF with reciprocal depression in other leads.

I.3.12 Posterior Infarction

- changes in lead V_1 (e.g. R wave, ST depression)
- occlusion of branches of right coronary artery

I.3.13 Chronic Myocardial Ischaemia

Reduced oxygen supply to muscle:

- ST depression
- T wave inversion
- occasionally tall pointed T wave

These changes can also occur during an exercise tolerance test when ischaemia develops (Figure I.22).

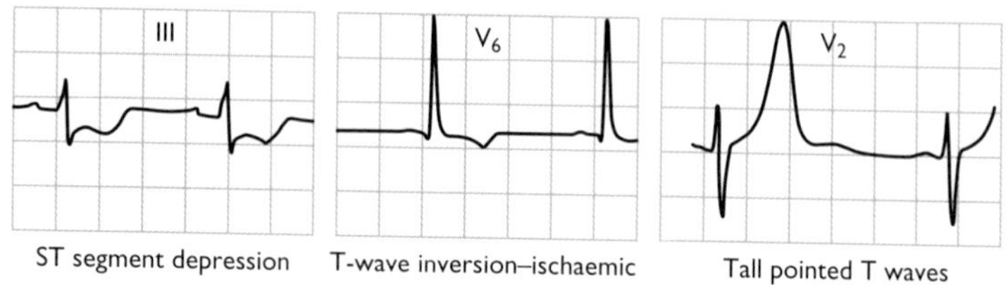

Figure I.22 Chronic myocardial ischaemia.

I.4 QRS Axis

- The direction of depolarization of the heart is sometimes helpful in diagnosis.
- Note that the axis deviation on its own is rarely significant but alerts you to look for right or left ventricular hypertrophy.
- Look at the standard leads for the most equiphasic QRS complex (R and S equal). The axis is approximately at right angles to this in the direction of the most positive standard lead (largest R wave) (Figure I.23).

I.4.1 Pattern Recognition

I.4.1.1 Left Axis Deviation

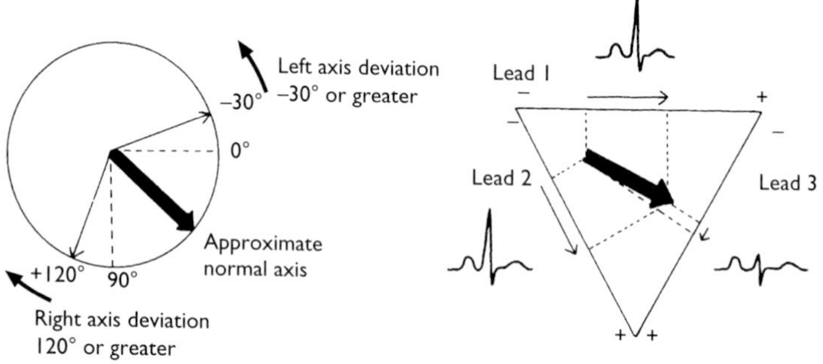

Figure I.23 QRS axis.

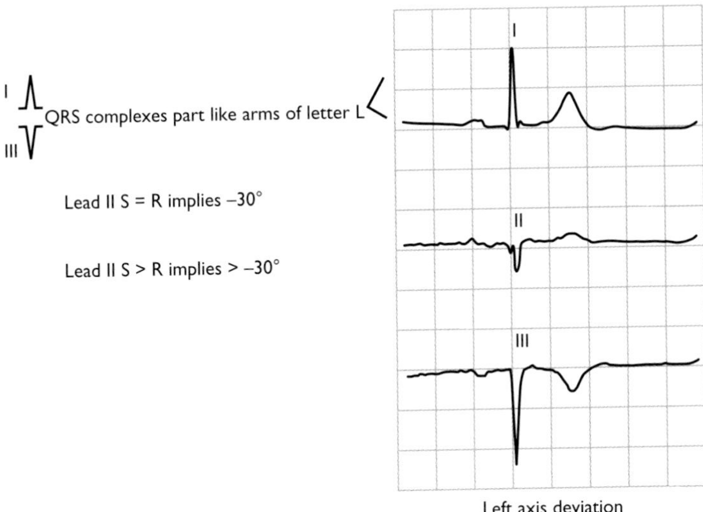

Figure I.24 Left axis deviation.

I.4.1.2 Right Axis Deviation

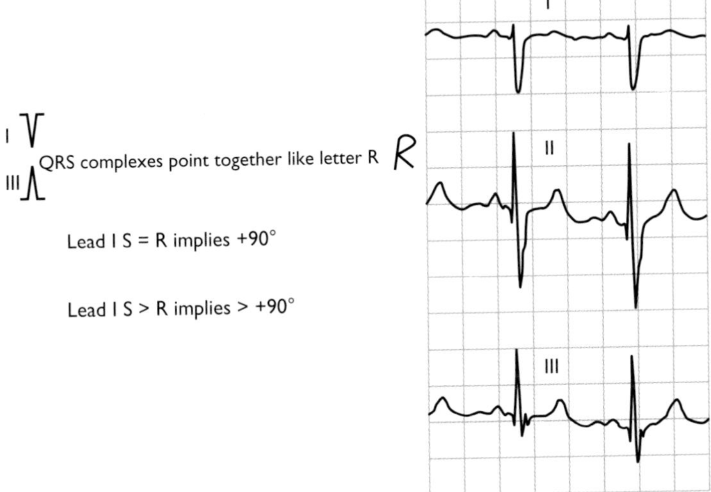

Figure I.25 Right axis deviation.

I.5 QRS Complex

- Normal if width < 0.12 second (three small squares).
- If > 0.12 second – bundle branch block.
- An apparently wide QRS complex, <0.12 second wide – partial bundle branch block or interventricular conduction defect.
- Left bundle branch block (LBBB) is usually associated with some form of heart disease.
- RBBB is often a normal variation, especially in athletes. Immediately after a myocardial infarction, the development of RBBB may be serious.

I.5.1 Left Bundle Branch Block

- M pattern in V_6.
- Throughout ECG, slurred ST segment and T wave inversion opposite to major deflection of QRS.
- Lead V_6
  - depolarization of septal muscle from right bundle gives positive deflection
  - right heart depolarization gives negative deflection
  - left heart depolarization gives positive deflection (Figure I.26)

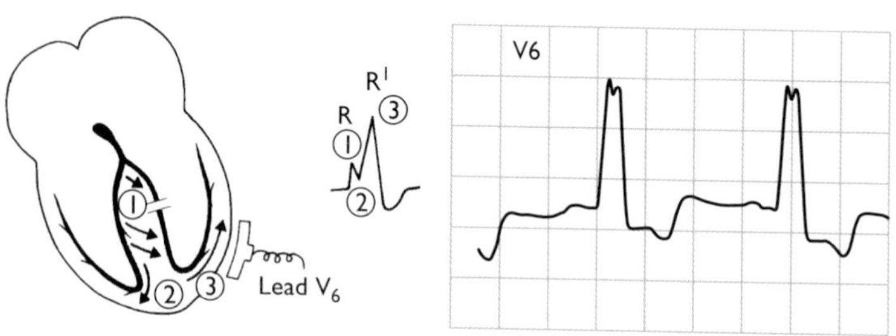

Figure I.26 Left bundle branch block.

- Standard leads
  - left axis deviation as impulse spreads from right bundle up to left ventricle
  - also occurs if only anterior fascicle of left bundle blocked
  - left anterior hemiblock

I.5.2 Right Bundle Branch Block

- M pattern in V_1.
- Lead V_1
  - depolarization of septal muscle from left bundle gives positive deflection
  - left heart depolarization gives negative deflection
  - right heart depolarization gives positive deflection (Figure I.27)
- Standard leads
  - axis usually normal, as depends on large muscle mass of left ventricle
  - if RBBB is associated with left axis, there is block of anterior fascicle of left bundle – bifascicular block

All heart is being excited via remaining posterior fascicle of left bundle.

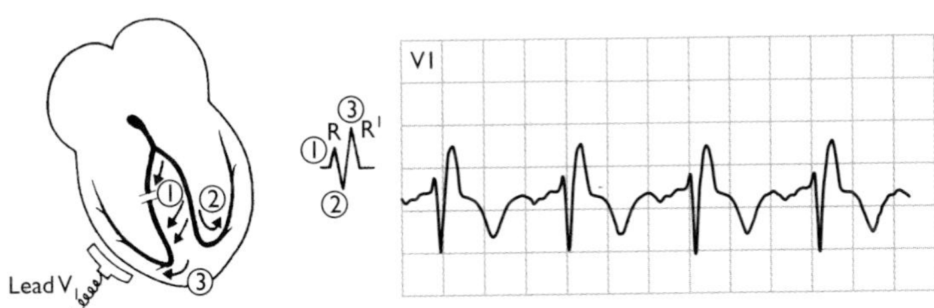

Figure I.27 Right bundle branch block.

I.6 Arrhythmias

- sinus arrhythmia
- ectopics
- tachycardias
- bradycardias

I.6.1 Sinus Arrhythmia

Normal variation with respiratory rate – increased rate on inspiration (Figure I.28).

I.7 Ectopics

I.7.1 Atrial Ectopics

Ectopic focus anywhere in atria. Depolarization spreads across atrium to AV node like any normal beat:

- P wave is abnormal shape
- normal QRS complex

The atrial ectopic focus must fire early or would be entrained by normal excitation:

- appears early on rhythm strip
- followed by compensatory pause – waiting for normal SA node cycle (Figure I.29)

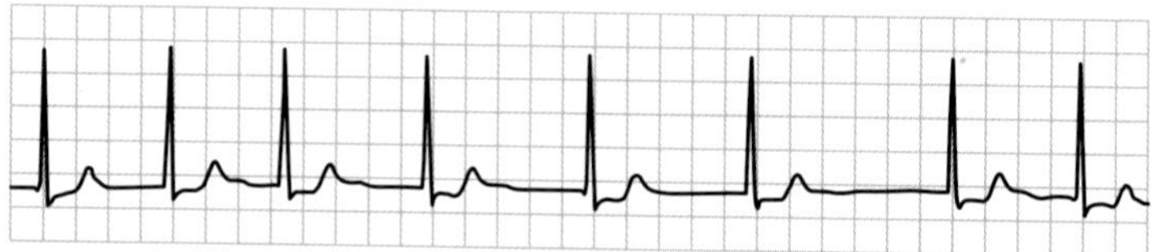

Figure I.28 Sinus arrhythmia.

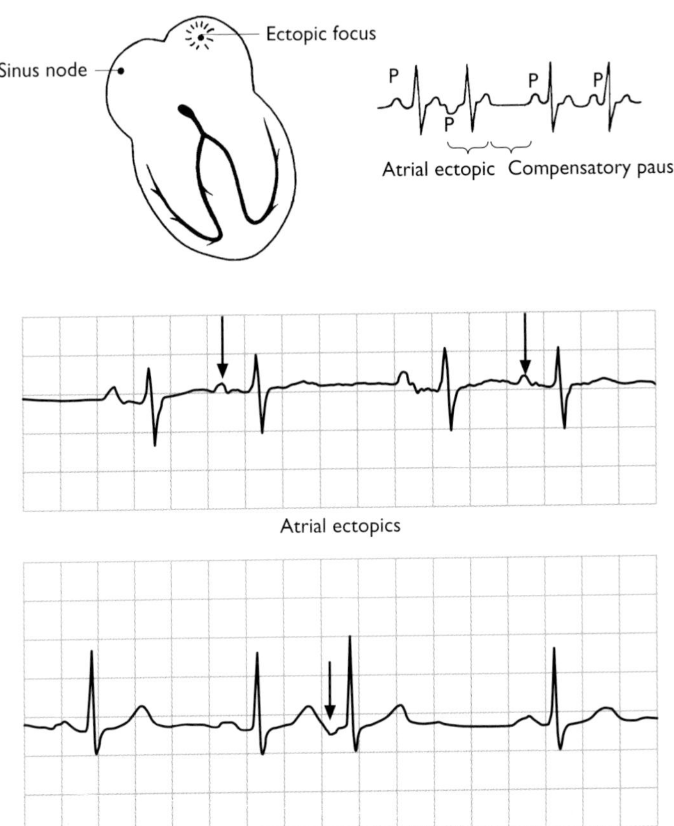

Figure I.29 Atrial ectopics.

I.7.2 Junctional or Nodal Ectopics

Ectopic at AV node; no P wave (Figure I.30).

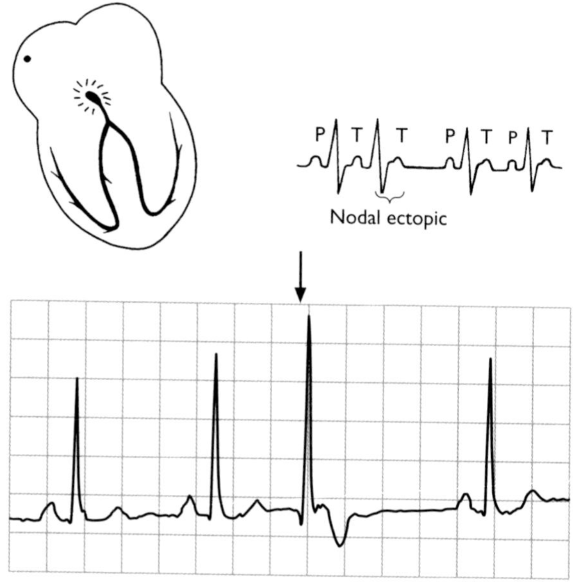

Figure I.30 Junctional or nodal ectopics.

I.7.3 Ventricular Ectopics

Ectopic anywhere in ventricles. Depolarization occurs first in that ventricle then spreads to other ventricle:

- no P wave
- wide complex
  - bundle branch block pattern
  - left focus – RBBB pattern
  - right focus – LBBB pattern

Atrial and junctional ectopics are invariably innocent when picked up on a random ECG. The majority of ventricular ectopics are also innocent except after a myocardial infarction. Ventricular ectopics picked up on routine monitoring of healthy patients are approximately proportional to age, i.e. 30% of 30-year-olds, 50% of 50-year-olds and almost

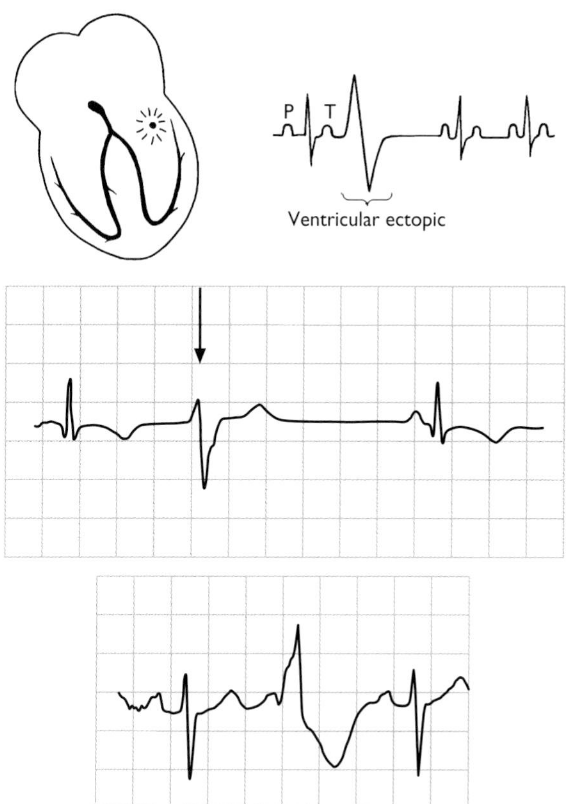

Figure I.31 Ventricular ectopics.

100% of 70-year-olds. Innocent ventricular ectopics usually disappear on exercise (Figure I.31).

I.8 Tachycardias

I.8.1 Classification of Tachycardias

- Tachycardias are divided into:
  - **narrow-complex regular** – QRS complex up to 0.08 second – two little squares on ECG
  - sinus tachycardia (Figure I.32)

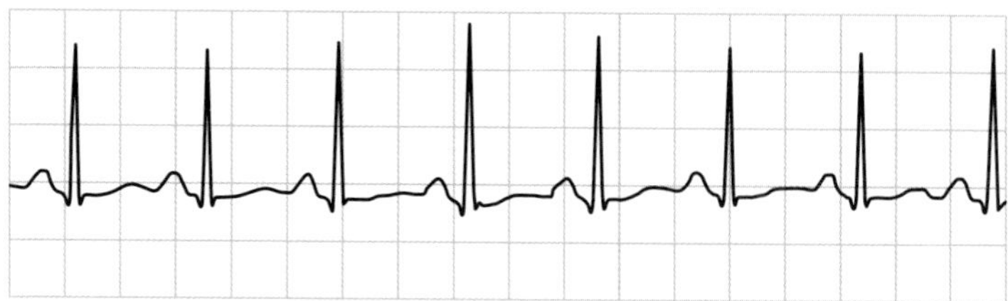

Figure I.32 Sinus tachycardia.

- supraventricular tachycardia, atrial tachycardia, atrial flutter
- narrow-complex irregular
- atrial tachycardia with varying block, atrial fibrillation
- **broad-complex** – QRS complex about 0.12 second – three small squares
- ventricular arrhythmias and occasionally supraventricular with aberrant (delayed) conduction

- Deciding whether a tachycardia is **atrial** or **ventricular** is not easy. Here are some pointers.
    - Narrow-complex tachycardias are usually atrial and broad-complex usually ventricular, **but not always**.
    - When acute ischaemic heart disease is present, tachycardias are usually ventricular. In the absence of ischaemic heart disease tachy- cardias are usually atrial, **but not always**.
    - If there is independent atrial activity (random appearance of p values), the tachycardia is ventricular.
    - Look at the patient's preceding ECGs or rhythm strip. If the tachycardia looks like a previous ectopic beat in shape, it will be that type of tachycardia.

- Vagal stimulation (rubbing carotid, etc.) will only be effective in atrial rhythms.
- The regularity or irregularity is not helpful in distinguishing ventricular from atrial arrhythmias.

I.8.2 Atrial Fibrillation

The electrical impulse and contraction travel randomly around the atria:

- 'bag-of-worms' quivering atria
- irregular little waves on ECG – best seen V_1 (Figure I.33).

When it first develops, often 150+, fibrillation waves are difficult to see:

- AV node fires irregularly
- normal QRS complexes
  If irregular rate, no P waves, normal QRS – likely to be atrial fibrillation.

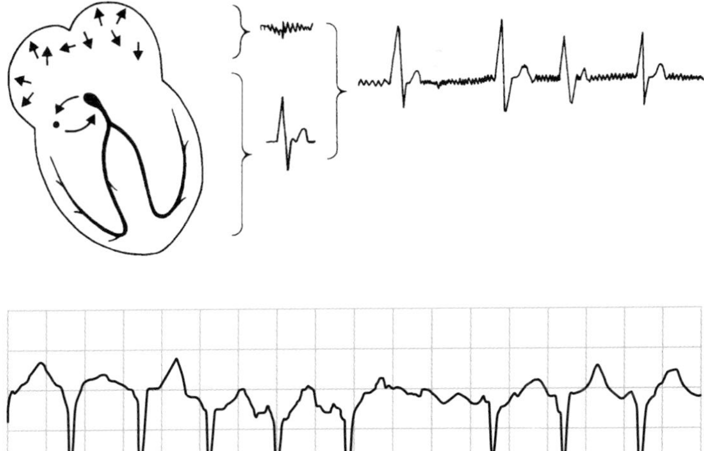

Figure I.33 Atrial fibrillation.

Digoxin is still the drug of choice – it decreases transmission of impulses down the bundle of His.

I.8.3 Atrial Flutter

Atria contract very rapidly, 200–250 beats min^{-1}, giving a sawtooth pattern, but the ventricles only respond to every second or third or fourth contraction (2 : 1, 3 : 1, 4 : 1 block) (Figure I.34).

Treated with digoxin, normally changes to atrial fibrillation.

I.8.4 Supraventricular Tachycardia (SVT)

- Arises near AV node, 170 beats min^{-1} or more, regular.
- Complexes are identical, normal width or wide if also bundle branch block.
- Common in young patients (20–30 years).

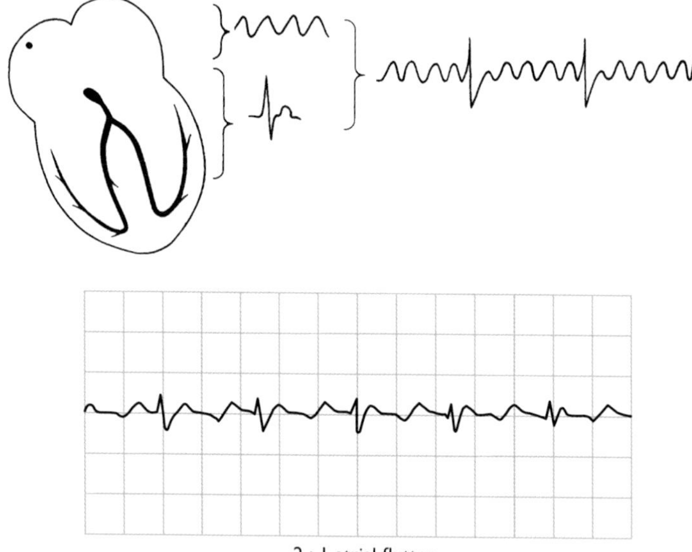

Figure I.34 Atrial flutter.

- Rarely represents heart disease.
- Sudden onset and finish.
- Last few minutes to several hours.
- Patient may be tired, light-headed, uncomfortable.
- In older patients supraventricular tachycardia (SVTs) more likely to represent heart disease (Figure I.35).

Vagal stimulation (rubbing carotid sinus) can terminate attack.

Re-entry is the most common mechanism for tachycardias (Figure I.36). Assumes two conduction pathways lead to ventricles. Normally conduction passes equally quickly down both pathways.

Problems arise when one pathway recovers more slowly than the other. When this happens the next conduction passes down only one pathway.

Conduction subsequently passes retrogradely up the other pathway, which is no longer refractory. This pathway then

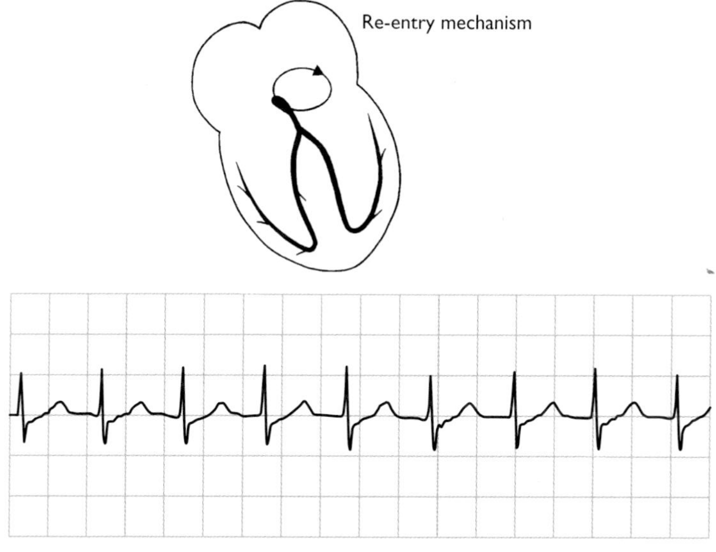

Figure I.35 Supraventricular tachycardia.

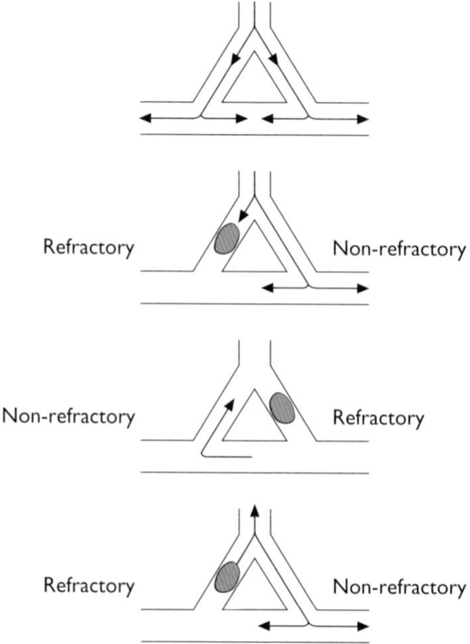

Figure I.36 The mechanism of re-entry tachycardias.

becomes refractory while the first pathway conducts again and the impulse races round the pathways to give a tachycardia.

I.8.5 Wolff–Parkinson–White Syndrome

This is the classic re-entry arrhythmia. There are two separate pathways from the atria to the ventricles. In the resting ECG the early entry, by the aberrant conduction pathway bypassing the bundle of His, is seen as a delta wave (Figure I.37).

I.8.6 Ventricular Tachycardia

- Potentially dangerous rhythm which can develop into ventricular fibrillation.

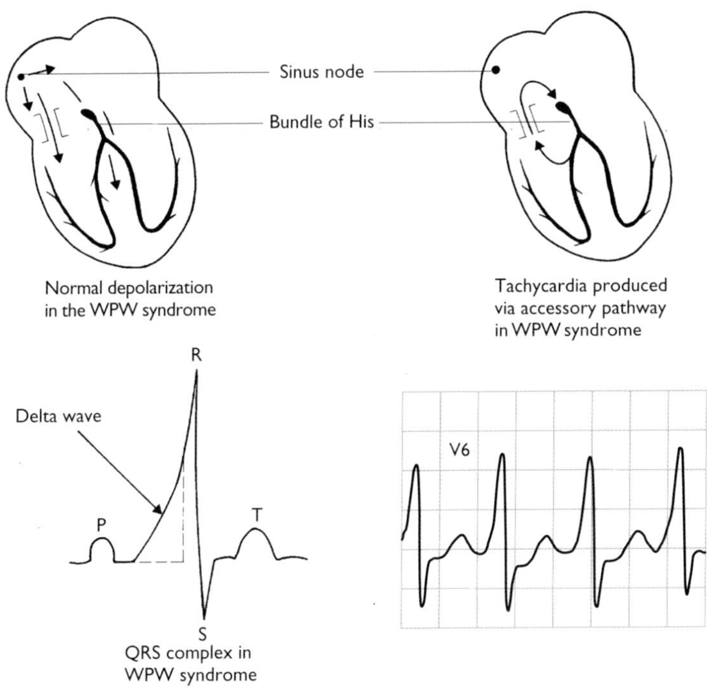

Figure I.37 Wolff–Parkinson–White syndrome.

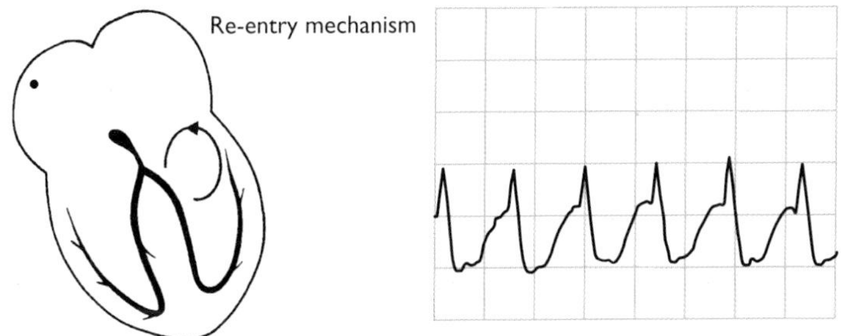

Figure I.38 Ventricular tachycardia.

- Rapid but not as fast as SVT (usually ·170 beats min^{-1}).
- Often slightly irregular.
- Patient often looks collapsed.

- Always wide QRS complex
    - LBBB pattern – right focus
    - RBBB pattern – left focus.

Treatment is with lidocaine 100 mg intravenously at once with transfer of the patient to hospital.

I.9 Bradycardias

Pulse rate < 60 beats min^{-1}.

I.9.1 Sinus

Normal P wave and QRS complexes.

- Causes:
    - athletic heart
    - β-blockers
    - hypothyroidism
    - raised intracranial pressure
    - pain with vagal response
        - dental pain
        - glaucoma
        - biliary colic (Figure I.40).

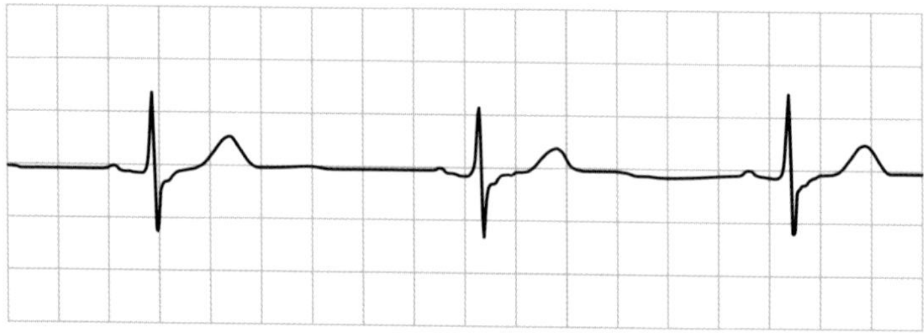

Figure I.39 Sinus bradycardia.

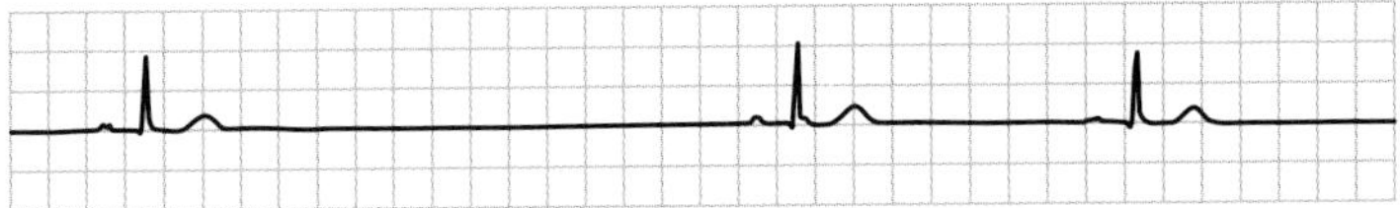

Figure I.40 Sinus arrest with vagal stimulation.

I.9.2 First-Degree Heart Block

- PR interval (beginning of P wave to beginning of QRS complex) >0.22 second (5.5 little squares).
- Depolarization delayed in the region of AV node (Figure I.41).

I.9.3 Wenckebach Heart Block

In a cycle of three or four beats, the PR interval gradually lengthens until a P wave appears on its own with no QRS complex. The cycle then repeats itself (Figure I.42).

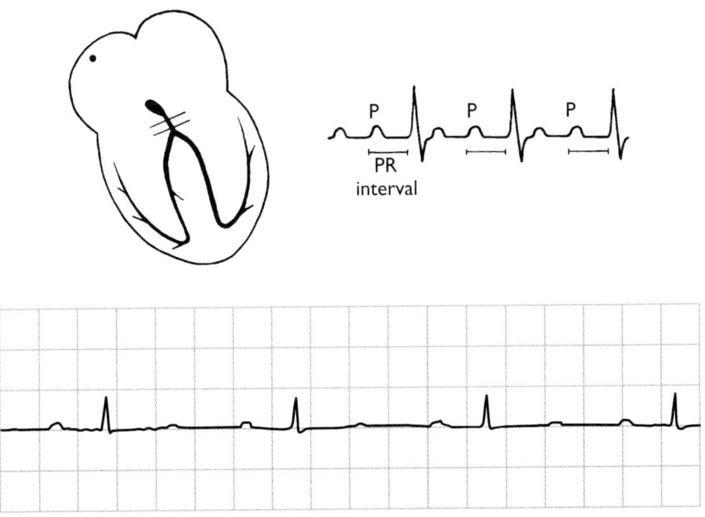

Figure I.41 First-degree heart block.

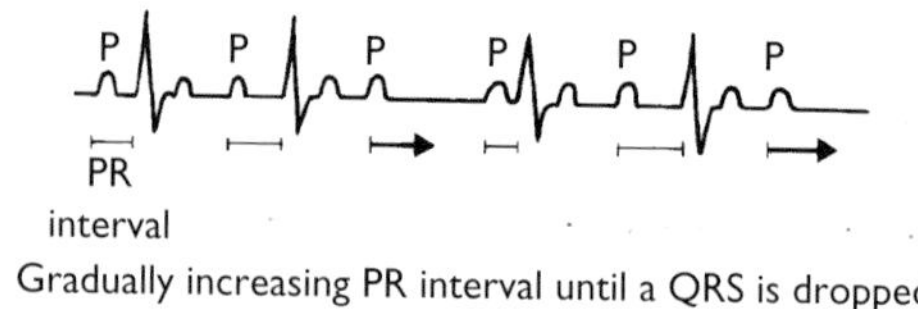

Figure I.42 Wenckebach heart block.

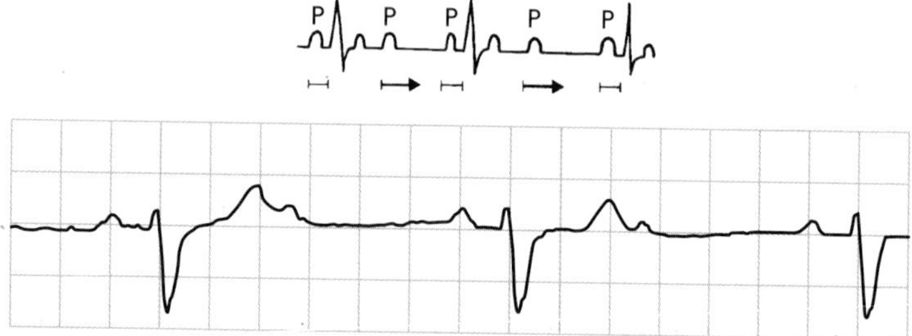

Figure I.43 2 : 1 block.

I.9.4 2:1 Block

The QRS complexes only respond to every other P wave, i.e. every other P wave has no QRS complex (Figure I.43).

I.9.5 Complete Heart Block

- No relation between P waves and QRS complex.
- Inherent ventricular rate about 40 beats min^{-1}.
- QRS complex abnormal as it arises in a ventricular focus (Figure I.44).

I.10 Pacemakers

- When conduction defects cause asystolic pauses or very slow heart rates, pacemakers can stimulate either the atrium or ventricle and restore rhythm.
- Pacemakers can be basic or very sophisticated.

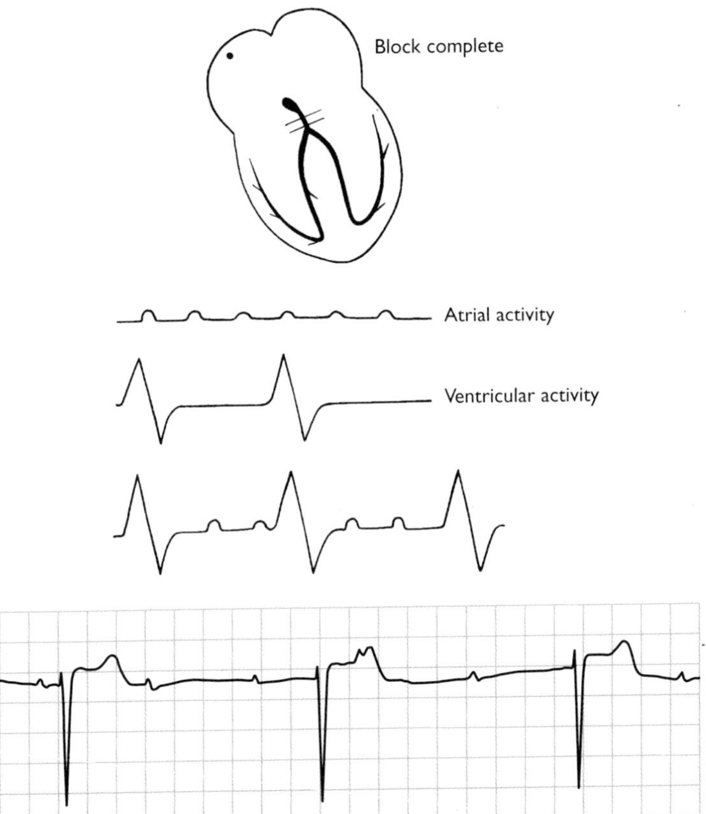

Figure I.44 Complete heart block.

I.10.1 Ventricle-Only Pacemakers

These are the most common type of pacemaker (80%+) (Figure I.45).

If the ventricle fails to produce an electrical signal (QRS complex), the pacemaker senses this and fires at approximately 60–70 beats min^{-1}. It is inhibited when the ventricle's QRS complex returns at an adequate rate.

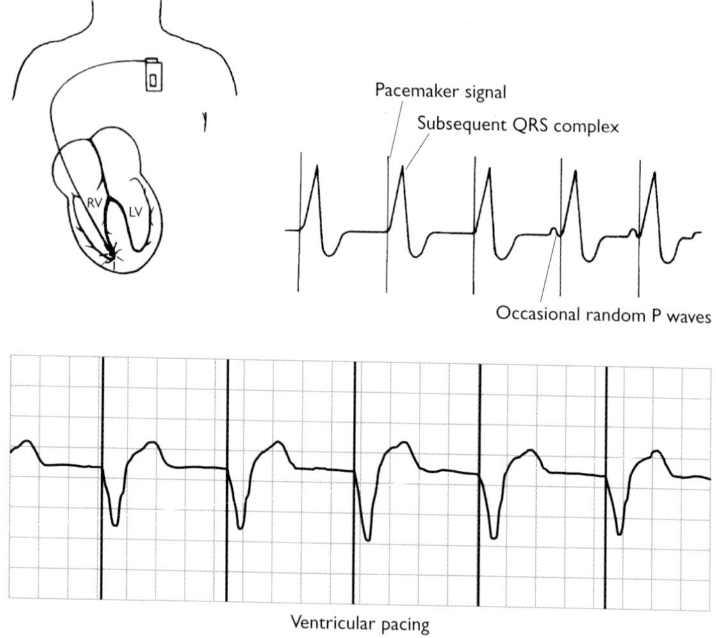

Figure I.45 Ventricle pacemakers.

I.10.2 Atrial-Only Pacemakers

In the sick sinus syndrome, the P wave fails to materialise but conduction in the AV node and bundle of His is normal. Pacing the atrium restores normal function.

I.10.3 Sequential Pacemakers

These pacemakers cause the sequential contraction of the atrium and ventricle in a more normal physiological way. This may provide a better cardiac output (Figure I.46).

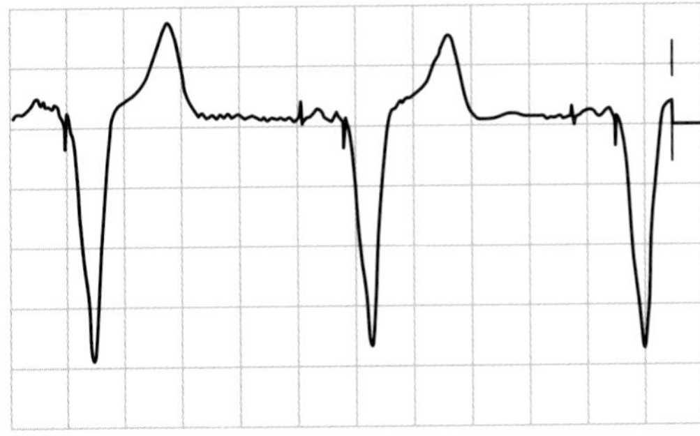

Figure I.46 Sequential pacing.

I.11 Looking at the ECG

Examine logically, reading complexes from left to right.

- Rhythm:
  - sinus rhythm ± ectopics; ignore sinus arrhythmia
  - regular
  - slow complete heart block
  - sinus bradycardia
  - fast sinus tachycardia
  - supraventricular tachycardia
  - ventricular tachycardia
  - regular atrial flutter
  - irregular
  - atrial fibrillation
  - atrial tachycardia with varying block
- **Rate:** add up the number of large squares between two successive beats. Divide into 300. For example:

$$\frac{300}{5 \text{ large squares}} = 60 \text{ beats/min}$$

1.5 squares	**= 200 beats min^{-1}**	**3.5**	**= 85 beats min^{-1}**
2	= 150 beats min^{-1}	4	= 75 beats min^{-1}
2.5	= 120 beats min^{-1}	5	= 60 beats min^{-1}
3	= 100 beats min^{-1}	6	= 50 beats min^{-1}

If the simple formula does not work for irregular rhythm then add up the number of complexes in six seconds (sometimes marked on the paper) and multiply by 10.

- **Complex shape** – brief guide:
    - P wave: abnormal shape
        - atrial ectopics, P mitrale, P pulmonale
    - 0.10–0.22 second (2.5–5.5 squares)
    - PR interval: prolonged
        - >0.22 second: first-degree heart block
        - <0.1 second: Wolff–Parkinson–White syndrome
    - QRS complex
        - large Q wave – full-thickness infarct?
        - wide QRS >0.12 second: branch block
        - R wave if large: ventricular hypertrophy?
- ST segment: elevated or depressed – ischaemia or other causes?
- T wave: if inverted – ischaemia or other causes?

In summary, particularly look for:

- abnormal rhythm
- abnormal rate
- abnormal QRS – especially ischaemia, infarct, hypertrophy

Index

Page numbers in *italic* refer to figures.
Page numbers in **bold** refer to tables.

A

Pocket Guide to Physical Assessment, First Edition. Edited by Carol Lynn Cox.

B

D

E

Q

R

S

T

U